Answering THE CALL

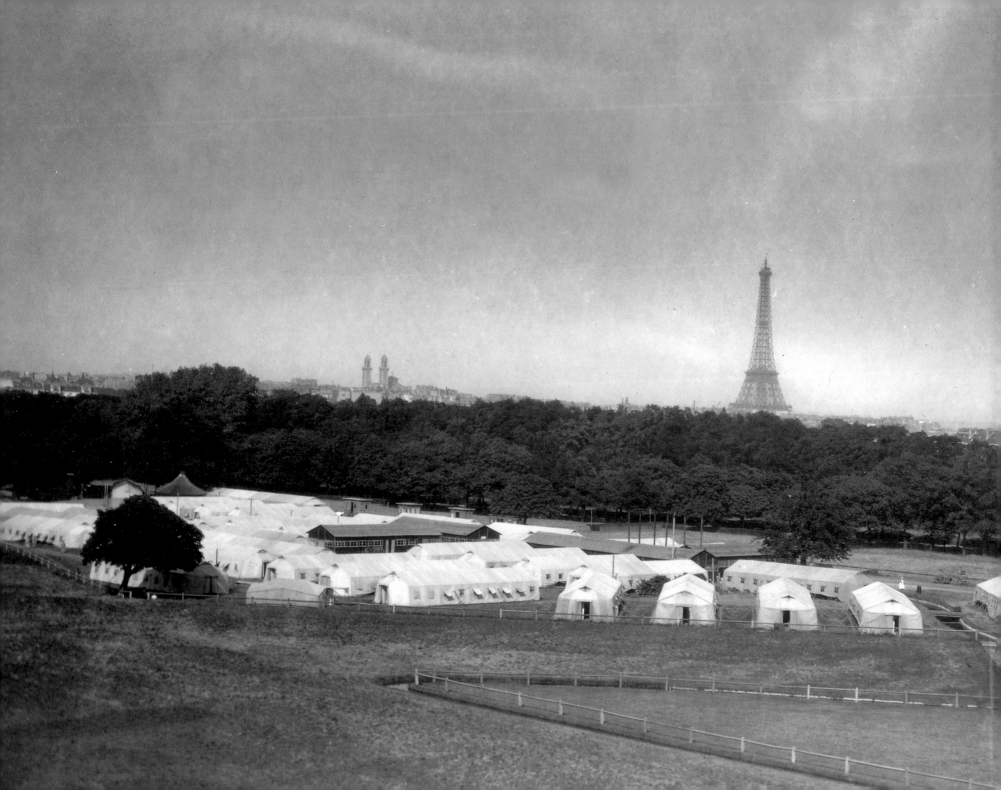

Answering THE CALL

THE U.S. ARMY NURSE CORPS, 1917–1919

A Commemorative Tribute to Military Nursing in World War I

Edited by

LISA M. BUDREAU, DPhil, MA and
RICHARD M. PRIOR, Lt. Col., Army Nurse Corps

Office of Medical History
OFFICE OF THE SURGEON GENERAL
United States Army, Falls Church, Virginia

Editorial Staff

Editor	Lisa M. Budreau, DPhil, MA
Co-Editor	Lt. Col. Richard M. Prior, USA
Creative Director/Production Manager	Christine Gamboa-Onrubia, MBA, Fineline Graphics LLC
Senior Volume Editor	Joan Redding

Published by the Office of The Surgeon General, Department of the Army, United States of America
Borden Institute, Walter Reed Army Medical Center, Washington, DC 20307-5001

Library of Congress Cataloging-in-Publication Data

Answering the call : the U.S. Army Nurse Corps, 1917-1919 : a
commemorative tribute to military nursing in World War I / edited by
Lisa M. Budreau and Richard M. Prior.
        p. cm.
1. World War, 1914–1918—Medical care—United States. 2. United
 States. Army Nurse Corps—History. 3. Military nursing—United
 States—History—20th century. I. Budreau, Lisa M. (Lisa Mary), 1957-
 II. Prior, Richard M.

D629.U6A65 2008
940.4'75—dc22

                                    2008060150

Printed in the United States of America

15 14 13 12 11 10 09 08   10 9 8 7 6 5 4 3 2
First Printing

Photo opposite title page: Hospital tents at Mobile Hospital No. 2, Auteuil, Paris, July 1, 1918.

For sale by the Superintendent of Documents, U.S. Government Printing Office
Internet: bookstore.gpo.gov   Phone: toll free (866) 512-1800;   DC area (202) 512-1800
Fax: (202) 512-2104 Mail: Stop IDCC, Washington, DC 20402-0001

ISBN 978-0-16-081724-3

Contents

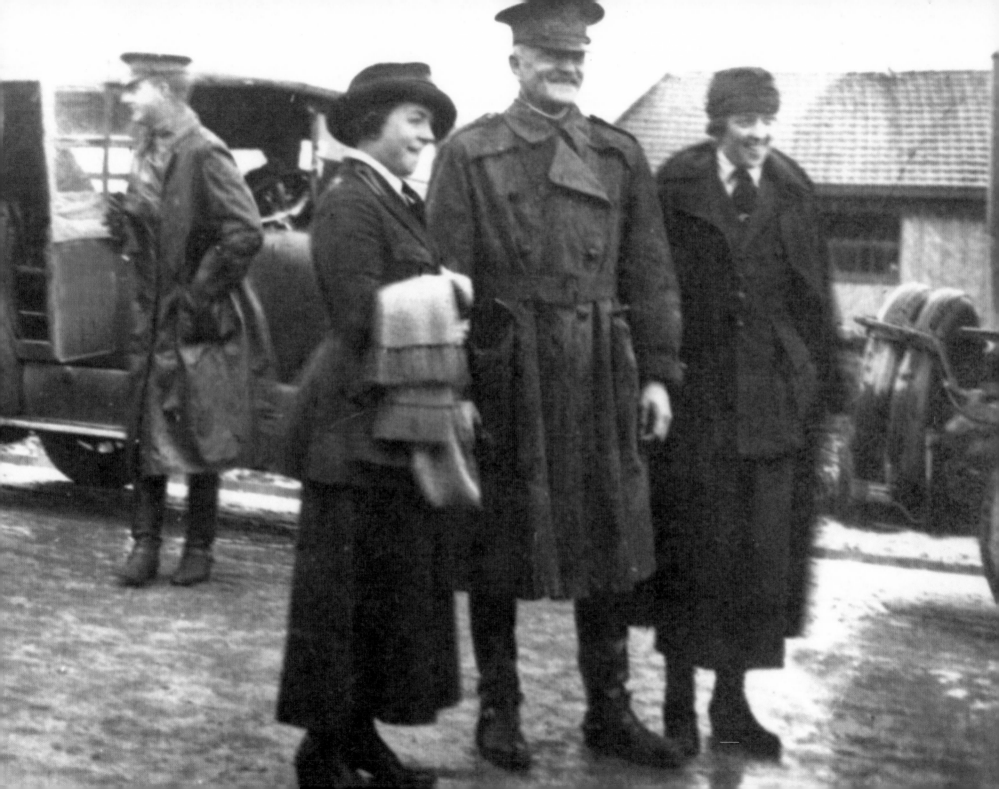

Foreword

ONLY SEVENTEEN YEARS AFTER THE ESTABLISHMENT of the Army Nurse Corps, America entered into a global conflict known as World War I. It was a short period for us, less than two years until the Armistice in 1918, but the demands on nurses were profound. During this period, the ANC grew from 403 members to over 22,000 utilizing a significant portion of all the professional nurses in the United States. Their willingness to volunteer was the blueprint for how nurses would answer the need across the 20th century when the patriots responded to a call to arms in support of our Nation and freedom around the world.

The contributions and accomplishments of World War I nurses advanced care of the wounded and ill across the world. They demonstrated the capabilities and importance of nurses on the front lines where their skills, dedication and compassion reduced morbidity and mortality of the battlefield. These achievements led to debate and progression on important issues to women and nurses for appropriate rank, compensation and retirement benefits. Through all of these challenges, Army Nurses focused on the needs of their patients and the mission clearly demonstrating that nurses were integral members of the healthcare team—long before the concept was accepted that care requires a team effort!

I ask that you ponder the strength and compassion of World War I Army nurses as you reflect on their stories, photos and experiences in this commemorative edition. They did not enjoy the technology that we now take for granted. However, their dedication to duty, commitment to all who needed their care, professionalism and patriotism set an incredible foundation for all of us who have followed their lead. I am grateful to these outstanding leaders and I know as you learn more about them, you will share my gratitude and amazement at all they contributed and achieved.

GALE S. POLLOCK
Major General, United States Army
Deputy Surgeon General for Force Management
Chief, Army Nurse Corps

(Opposite) *General John J. Pershing, Commander AEF, with Army nurses.*

THE YEAR 2008 MARKS THE 90TH ANNIVERSARY of the signing of the armistice that ended World War I on November 11, 1918. The extreme conditions of this bloody global conflict posed an unprecedented challenge to the U.S. Army's medical service, which grew increasingly reliant upon the support of its nursing volunteers. Women of the Army Nurse Corps (ANC) endured the hardships of battle while carving themselves a niche that included service in camp and field hospitals, evacuation hospitals, mobile hospitals, hospital trains, and base hospitals.

By mid-1918, the strength of the ANC had grown to more than 12,000 from just over 1,000 the year before. Recognition of the valuable role nurses played during the war led to the establishment, also in 1918, of the Army School of Nursing, a highly respected and unique institution that set exacting and enduring standards of quality.

In dedicating this commemorative publication to all Army nurses who served during the First World War, the Office of The Surgeon General and the U.S. Army Medical Command pay tribute to the significant contributions that the Army Nurse Corps made to the advancement of military medicine 90 years ago.

(Opposite) *Changing dressings at Base Hospital No. 52, Rimaucourt, Haute Marne, France.*

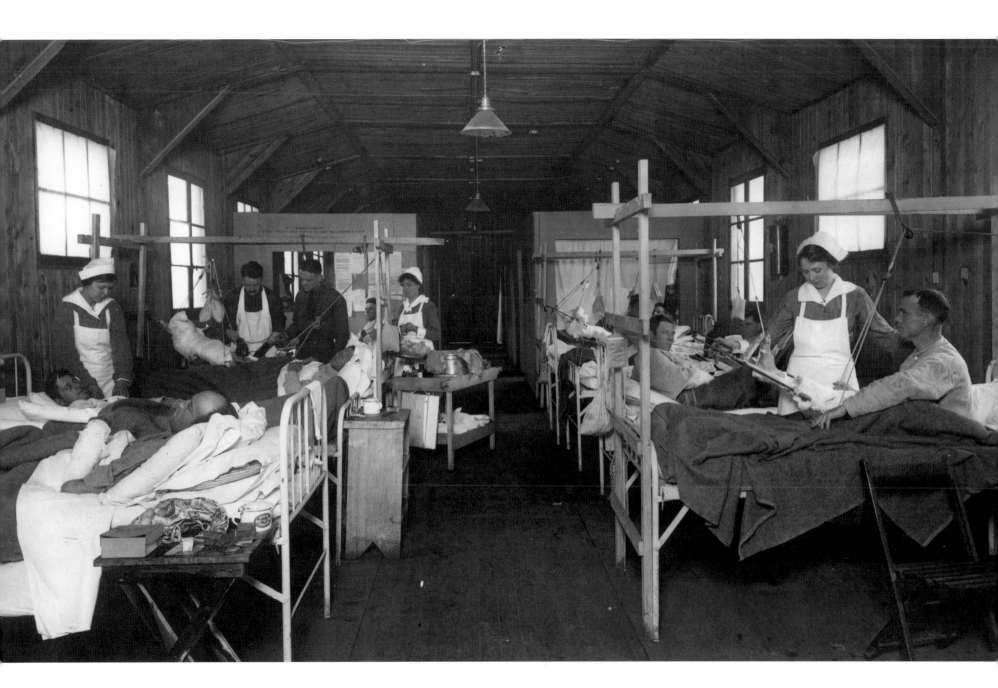

Sergeant First Class Clarence Jackson and Private First Class John Dadette, Signal Corps Photographers, 33rd Division, Luxembourg.

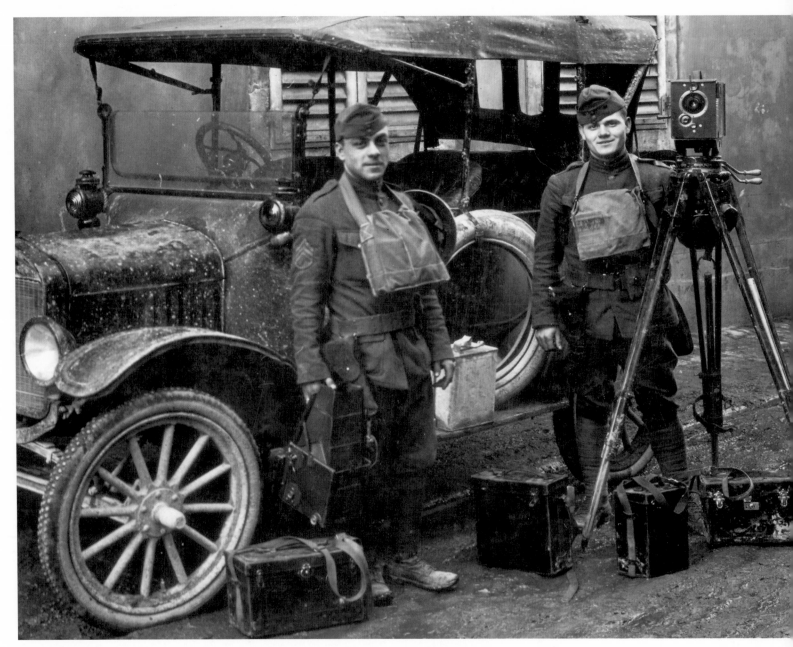

Editor's Note

GATHERED HERE FOR THE FIRST TIME is a rare and carefully chosen collection that depicts the rich and varied experiences of Army nurses during the First World War as recorded by U.S. Army Signal Corps photographers. Thanks to their diligent efforts, we have inherited a priceless legacy of the war as seen through their lens.

Although these images appear in various tones of black and white, they are embedded with the ever-changing hues of human drama, emotion, tragedy, and exhilaration that typically color the personal wartime experience.

To accompany this photographic anthology, I have selected numerous excerpts from contemporary historians whose well-researched accounts of the ANC in 1918 offer invaluable understanding of the role these brave volunteers played. Included among these are Lettie Gavin's *American Women in World War I* (1997); *A History of the U.S. Army Nurse Corps* by Mary T. Sarnecky (1999); and *Heritage of Leadership, Army Nurse Corps Biographies* by Dorothy B. Pocklington (2004).

The earlier writings of Julia Stimson, the indefatigable Superintendent of the Army Nurse Corps in 1918, are also represented here as they appeared in her printed wartime letters *Finding Themselves* (1918) and "The Army Nurse Corps" section of *The Medical Department of the United States Army in the World War* (1927). *The Annual Report of The Surgeon General, 1919*, also provided a wealth of practical data, but my deepest gratitude is reserved for those women who left behind a trove of first-hand accounts in their personal diaries and letters home. These often amusing, occasionally distressing, and frequently heartrending voices vividly animate the extraordinary tale depicted on the following pages.

LISA M. BUDREAU, DPhil, MA, Editor
Office of Medical History
Office of The Surgeon General
Falls Church, Virginia

Preface

THE EVOLUTIONARY HISTORY OF THE ARMY NURSE CORPS is perhaps the most unusual of all the Army officer corps. The Corps was not established with military rank and structure, but began in 1901 with barely more than 100 female nurses who lacked appropriate titles, military status, or even uniforms. Each progressive step in the organization's history thereafter required a series of victories, each built upon previous successes.

World War I nurses were highly instrumental in this developmental process, despite the frequent hardships and danger many faced. They were the first to prove that nurses held a rightful place at the front lines, where they could make a valuable, often life-saving difference. In so doing, these were the first women to receive recognition for gallantry on the battlefield. Because of their performance, after World War I a rudimentary rank structure and retirement allocation for all members of the Army Nurse Corps were enacted.

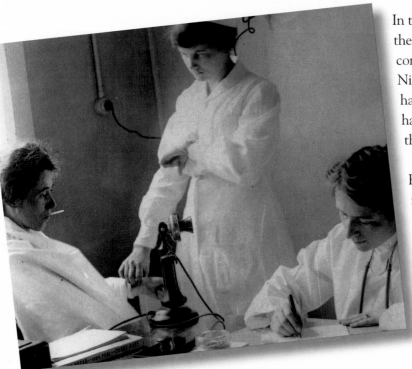

In these pages you will see the faces of the very people responsible for the Corps' earliest achievements as depicted in photographs, often accompanied by their own words. Quite simply, they changed our history. Ninety years later, Army nurses have risen to new heights. Now, they have the opportunity to be board-selected for command positions and have even risen to conquer such monumental challenges as serving as the acting Surgeon General of the United States Army.

Fortunately, the history of the Army Nurse Corps also attracts the interest of scholars external to the organization. I would like to thank Gray & Associates Consultants for supporting this project and Dr. Lisa Budreau for her interest, immense skill, and determination in seeing that this wonderful story is told.

LT. COL. RICHARD M. PRIOR, USA
Army Nurse Corps Historian, 2006–2008

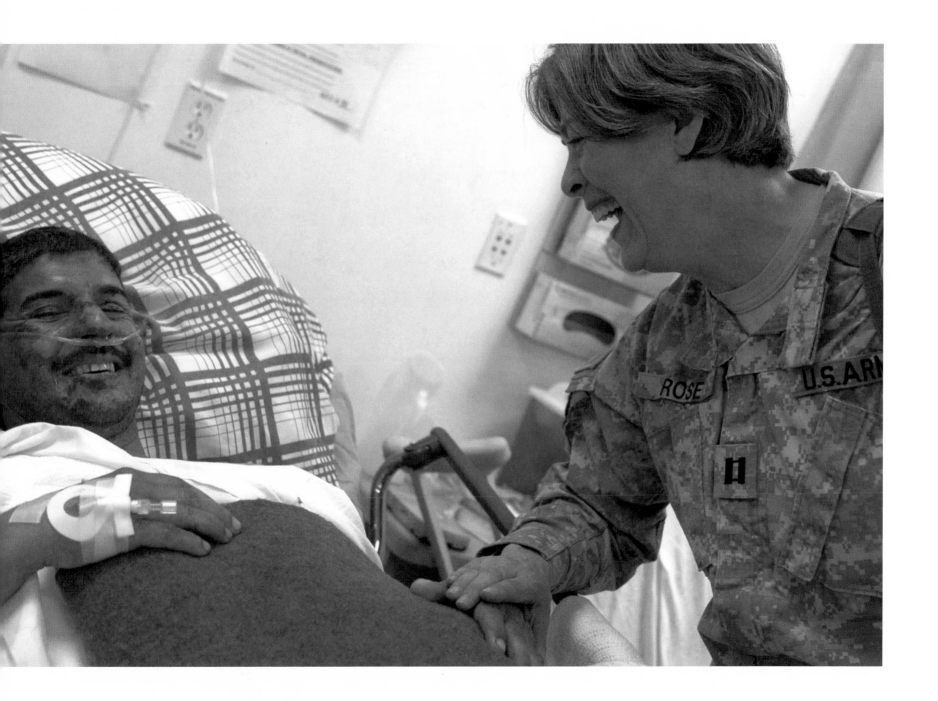

Some of America's best uniformed World War I artists, such as Captain Harvey Dunn, Captain Wallace Morgan, and Captain George Matthews Harding, illustrated the combat scenes featured herein. Harding was one of the few artists who used a camera in addition to sketches and notes to record his impressions in the field. The U.S. Army Signal Corps later photographed his work, now part of the National Archives' still photograph collection.

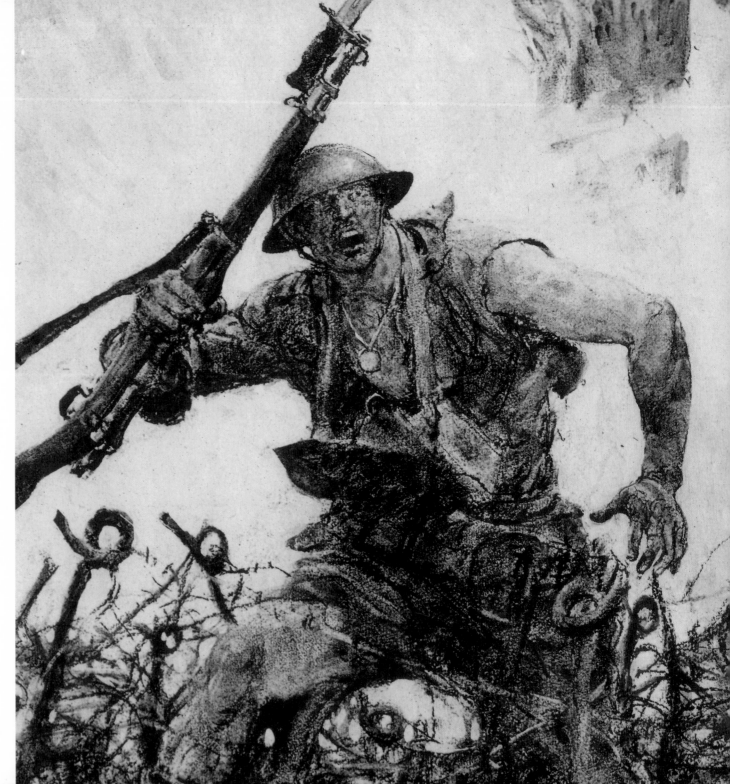

Introduction

THE FIRST WORLD WAR, a global military conflict that took place primarily in Europe from August 4, 1914, to November 11, 1918, resulted chiefly from the breakdown of old alliances among European powers. The Entente was comprised of France, Russia (until 1917), Great Britain, and later Italy (from 1915). The United States entered the conflict when it declared war on Germany on April 6, 1917, as an "associate" to the Allied nations. Together, they defeated the Central Powers of the Austro-Hungarian, German, and Ottoman empires.

The conflagration, characterized by trench warfare, machine guns, barbed wire, shell holes, widespread chemical warfare, and masses of artillery, was responsible for the death of approximately 9 million people worldwide. Often called the "Great War," these years of bloody conflict had a devastating impact on the history of the 20th century. Millions of individuals suffered fatal or often disabling wounds and injuries, and each belligerent nation bore immeasurable and long-term social, financial, and psychological costs.

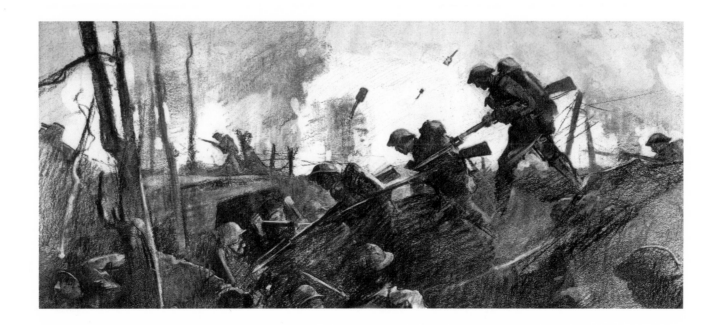

The Army Nurse Corps

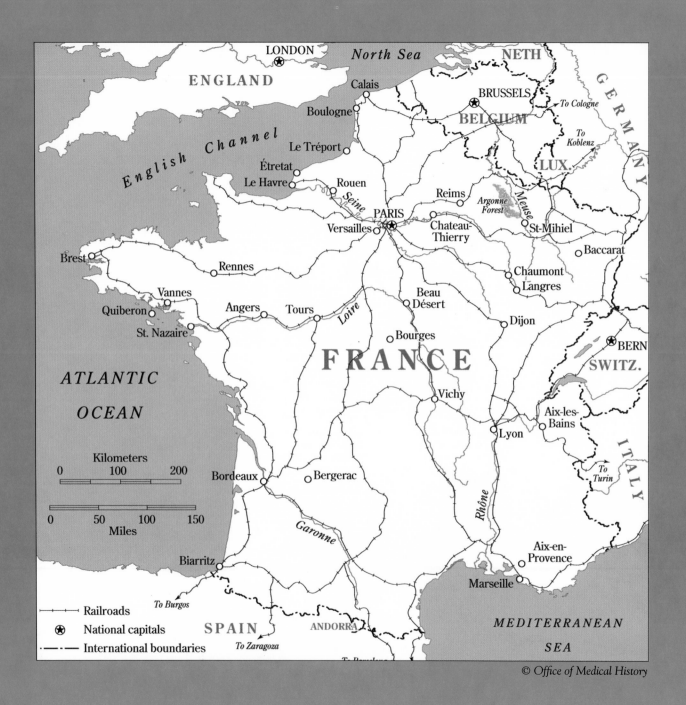

Historical Background

WHEN THE UNITED STATES ENTERED THE WAR in Europe in April 1917, almost three years after it began, the Army Medical Department was better prepared for war than ever before, but its preparation fell short of the demands that lay ahead. Initially, the department was unable to answer the call for medical assistance from Britain, a nation that had been at war since 1914.

The War Department had begun a reorganization of the Army's Medical Department on February 2, 1901, that included the creation of an Army Nurse Corps of trained female nurses, responsible for the care of sick and wounded soldiers. This action freed the enlisted men of the Hospital Corps to fill positions in field medical units and hospitals as well as in infantry and cavalry regiments, thus improving the quality and efficiency of military medical care.

Jane Delano, who had first become involved with the Red Cross as a volunteer nurse during the Spanish-American War, was appointed the second Superintendent of the Army Nurse Corps in 1909. She was also named chairman of the National Committee on Red Cross Nursing Service that same year. Delano began developing the Red Cross Nursing Service and recruited a growing list of volunteers who could later enroll as either an Army or Red Cross nurse. In 1912 she resigned her position as Superintendent to focus solely on the Red Cross, a move that strengthened the affiliation between the Nurse Corps and the American Red Cross.

Despite the continued growth of the Medical Department, no regular Army hospital units were yet ready for departure at the outbreak of World War I. However, a number of 500-bed Red Cross Army Base Hospital units were trained and ready for service. Six of these units (Base Hospital Nos. 2, 4, 5, 10, 12, and 21) were ordered to France in May 1917 to support the British Expeditionary Force.

Chief Nurses

"CHIEF NURSES WERE NOT TO BE APPOINTED as such, but were to be selected by promotion from the grade of nurse. A chief nurse invariably was to be assigned to duty when two or more nurses were serving at the same station. On the other hand a chief nurse was not to be assigned to duty permanently, except by the Surgeon General, upon the recommendation of the superintendent of the Army Nurse Corps. Nor was a nurse to be assigned permanently to duty as chief nurse until after she had passed a satisfactory examination.

"Nurses who exhibited marked executive ability, good judgment, and tact were to be recommended to the Surgeon General by the commanding officer of a hospital or other Medical Department formation with which they were on duty for examination for promotion to the grade of chief nurse." (*The Medical Department of the US Army in the World War [hereafter, The Medical Dept in the World War], Vol. XIII, p. 288*)

"[W]ith the rapid opening of new camps and cantonments in 1917, and the assignment of nurses to the hospitals there, a great many chief nurses had to be appointed. In so far as it was possible to do so, candidates for chief nurseship were selected from women already in the corps, but during the earlier months of the war such a source of supply could not begin to meet the demand. Fortunately, hundreds of leaders in the nursing profession in civil life eagerly responded to the summons and entered the Army Nurse corps either directly or through the American Red Cross nursing service." (*The Medical Dept in the World War, Vol. XII, p. 295*)

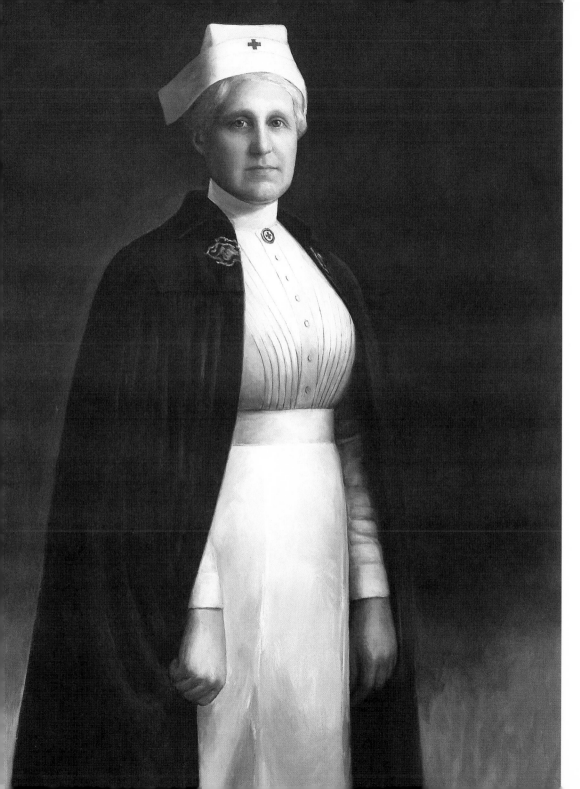

"When the Great War ended, Jane Delano, the stalwart of the Red Cross, could look back on her almost superhuman efforts, which included the registration of 18,989 graduate nurses for Army, Navy, and Red Cross service during the war." (GAVIN, P. 62)

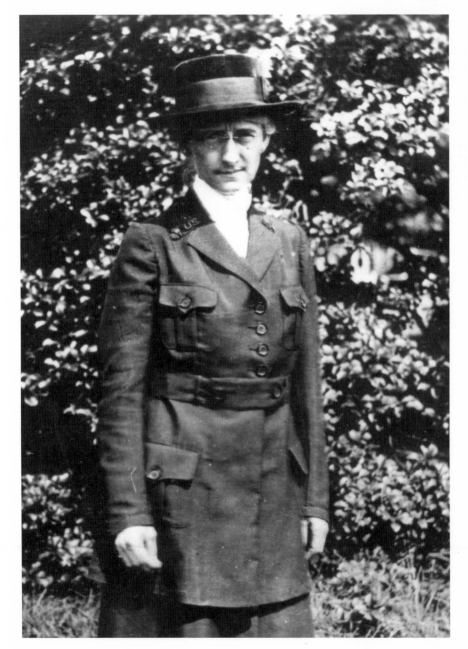
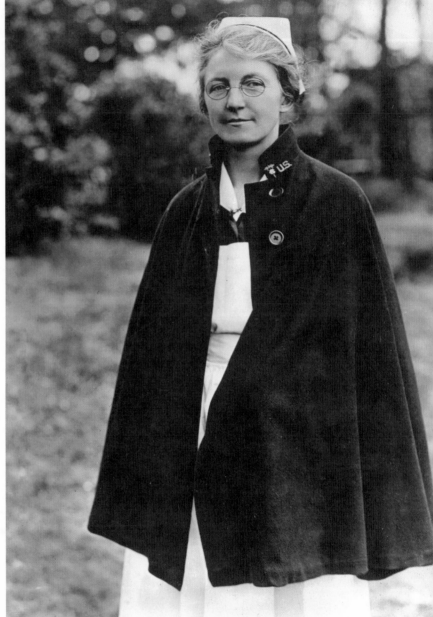

In 1914, Dora E. Thompson distinguished herself as the first regular Army nurse to become the Superintendent of the Army Nurse Corps, and the first Superintendent to lead the Corps during a war. She was also the first Superintendent to lead Army nurses under the organization's new title, Army Nurse Corps (ANC). Thompson entered the Army one year after the Nurse Corps was authorized by an act of Congress on February 2, 1901. The Corps she joined had only 100 nurses when it began, and no provision for awarding military rank to Army nurses existed at that time.

Thompson once told an audience that the creation of the Nurse Corps had been a "rather up hill battle" and that they received much opposition, as many people thought women were not suited for work in Army hospitals. Moreover, they believed female nurses would be more of a burden than a help.

Under her leadership, the ANC grew from less than 400 to 21,480 nurses serving in the United States, Europe, and the Philippines. She received the Distinguished Service Medal in November 1919. In December, 1919, Thompson resigned as Superintendent of the ANC, a post that Julia C. Stimson then assumed. Thompson died at age 77 in 1954 and was buried at Arlington National Cemetery. *(Pocklington, pp. 25–29)*

(Opposite and Right)
Dora E. Thompson
(1876–1954)

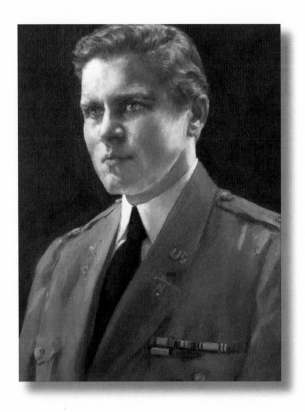

Julia C. Stimson (1881–1948) received her bachelor's degree from Vassar College in 1901. While considering the study of medicine, she completed graduate work in biology and medical drawing at Columbia University. She entered nurse training at New York Hospital in 1904. After graduating in 1908, Stimson served as superintendent of nurses at the newly-opened Harlem Hospital until 1911.

During World War I, Stimson sailed for Europe as chief nurse of the Red Cross Army Unit from Washington University, St. Louis, which became known as Base Hospital No. 21. She served in this post until April 1918, when she left to become head of the Red Cross Nursing Service in France and later Superintendent of the Army Nurse Corps (a title that changed to "Chief" during her tenure) in December 1919. She stayed in that position until 1937.

Julia Stimson was awarded the Distinguished Service Medal for her service in France. In 1920 she became the first woman to achieve the rank of major in the U.S. Army.

"We have had less than a week's notice to get ready for mobilization for service in France, and so it has been a rushing week. . . . Of course this order for foreign service is playing havoc with the personnel of the Unit, so few expected to be called for duty abroad. In fact, no one expected a call of this sort at all. I have been quite disgusted with the quitters who, for one reason or another, have begged to be excused. I have had about ten drop out, but I am finding substitutes who I think will be much more desirable than such weak-kneed individuals. I am to have a detachment of Kansas City nurses attached to my corps. . . . Two whose names I submitted I have had to drop by orders from Washington because they were born in Germany." *(May 4, 1917, Stimson, Finding Themselves)*

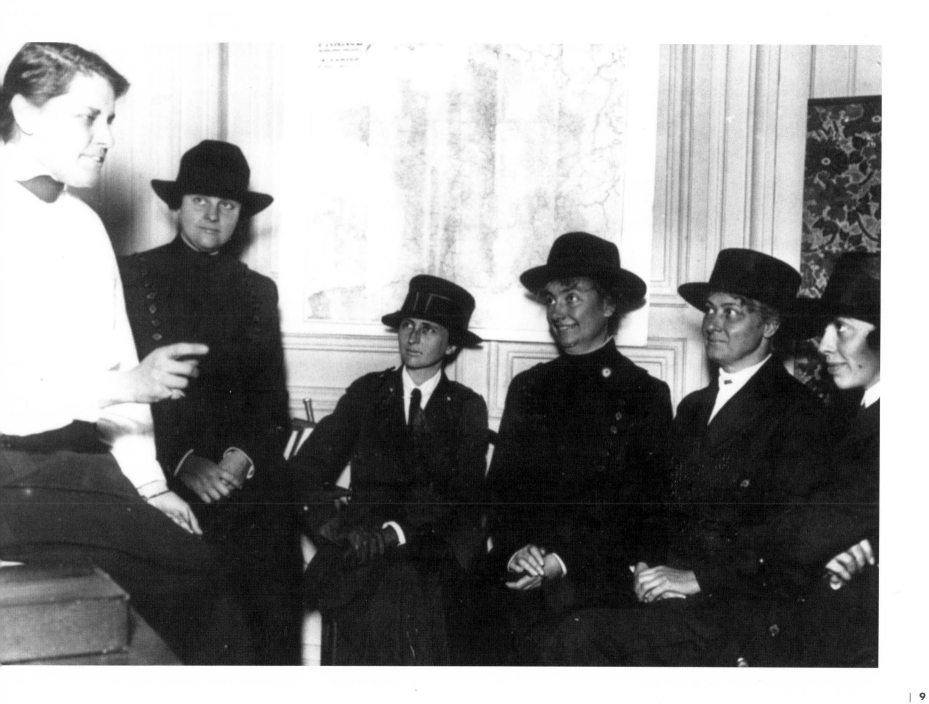

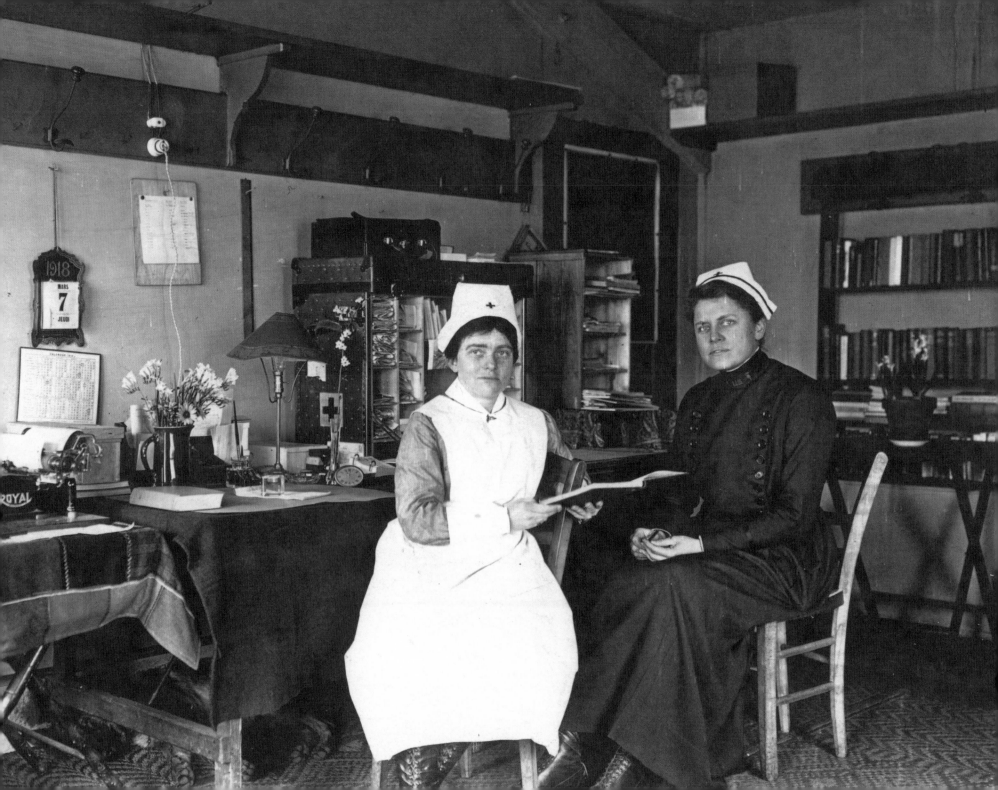

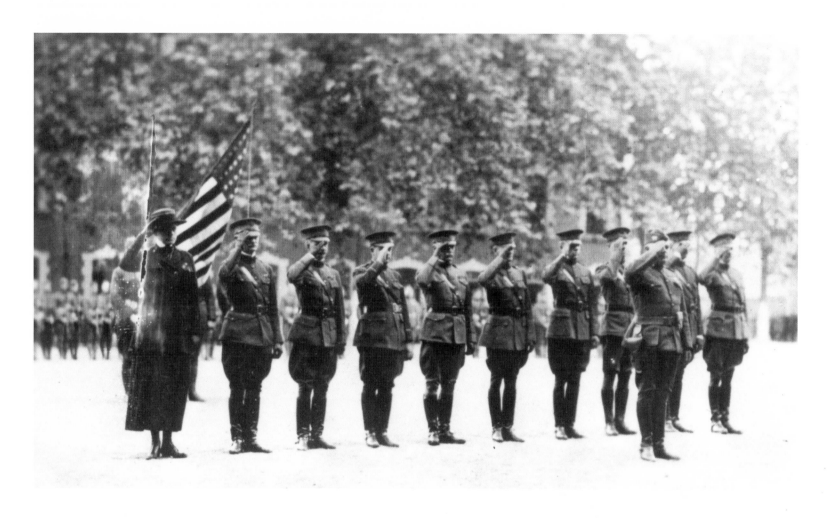

(Opposite) "*Miss Taylor and I are in our cozy office waiting for the time for the evening report. . . . We have both been to first supper and will now rest ourselves a little for this half hour. I wish you all could see how nice our office is. We have the tiniest coal stove that ever existed, and yet it is just the right size for this place. We have been having a fire in it for the past few days, for it has been very cold and raining almost every day.*" (OCTOBER 14, 1917, STIMSON, FINDING THEMSELVES)

(Above) *Julia Stimson in officer formation.*

Esther Voorhes Hasson was born in Baltimore, Maryland, on September 20, 1867. She was well educated and came from a family dedicated to military service: her father served as a surgeon during the Civil War and her brother graduated from the U.S. Naval Academy at Annapolis.

The Spanish-American War, which predated the establishment of the Army Nurse Corps by three years, required contract nurses to serve in the absence of an established military nurse corps. Hasson supported the war as one of six contract nurses who sailed on the maiden voyage of the Army hospital ship *Relief* in July 1898.

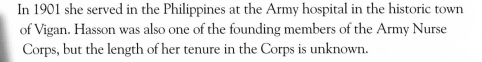

In 1901 she served in the Philippines at the Army hospital in the historic town of Vigan. Hasson was also one of the founding members of the Army Nurse Corps, but the length of her tenure in the Corps is unknown.

In 1908 the Navy Nurse Corps was founded and quickly received a suitable Superintendent. Hasson was one of three women who applied for the position. She was selected and appointed on August 18, 1908, at the age of 41, by Navy Surgeon General Admiral P.M. Rixey. In 1910 Hasson began having personal disagreements with the new Navy Surgeon General, Admiral C.F. Stokes, and by 1911 she could no longer tolerate the vitriolic working conditions and resigned.

After leaving the Navy, Hasson reentered the Army Nurse Corps through the reserves. She was activated when the United States entered World War I and assigned to Base Hospital No. 12, then Army Red Cross Hospital No. 1 and Provisional Base Hospital No. 1. She was awarded the French *Medal d'Honneur des Epidemics* for her performance in the war. Hasson died in Washington, D.C., on March 8, 1942. *(Photograph courtesy of Navy Bureau of Medicine and Surgery Archives)*

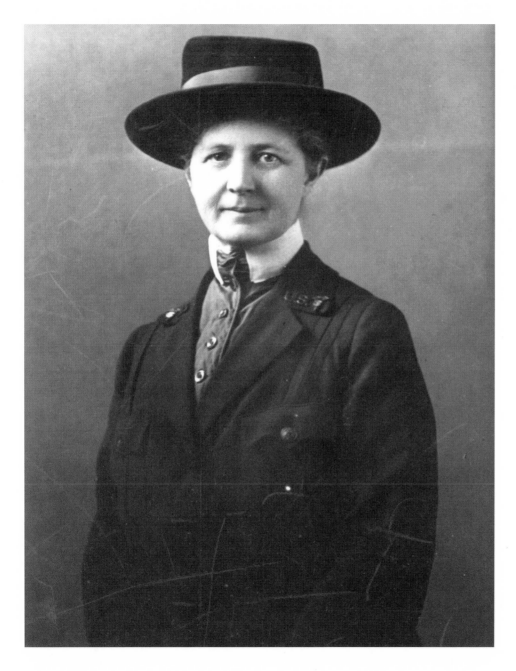

Chief Nurse Vashti Bartlett (1873–1969) was a 1906 graduate of Johns Hopkins University. Her nursing career included service in Labrador, Newfoundland, Siberia, and Haiti, but from March 1915 to January 1916, she served with the American Red Cross in France and Belgium. From March 1917 to August 13, 1918, Bartlett served as Clara Noyes' assistant in the Department of Nursing, Bureau of Field Nursing Service, at Red Cross Headquarters in Washington, D.C. Then, in August 1918, she returned to France to serve with the ANC as Chief Nurse of Base Hospital No. 71 until April 1919.

The Red Cross Solution

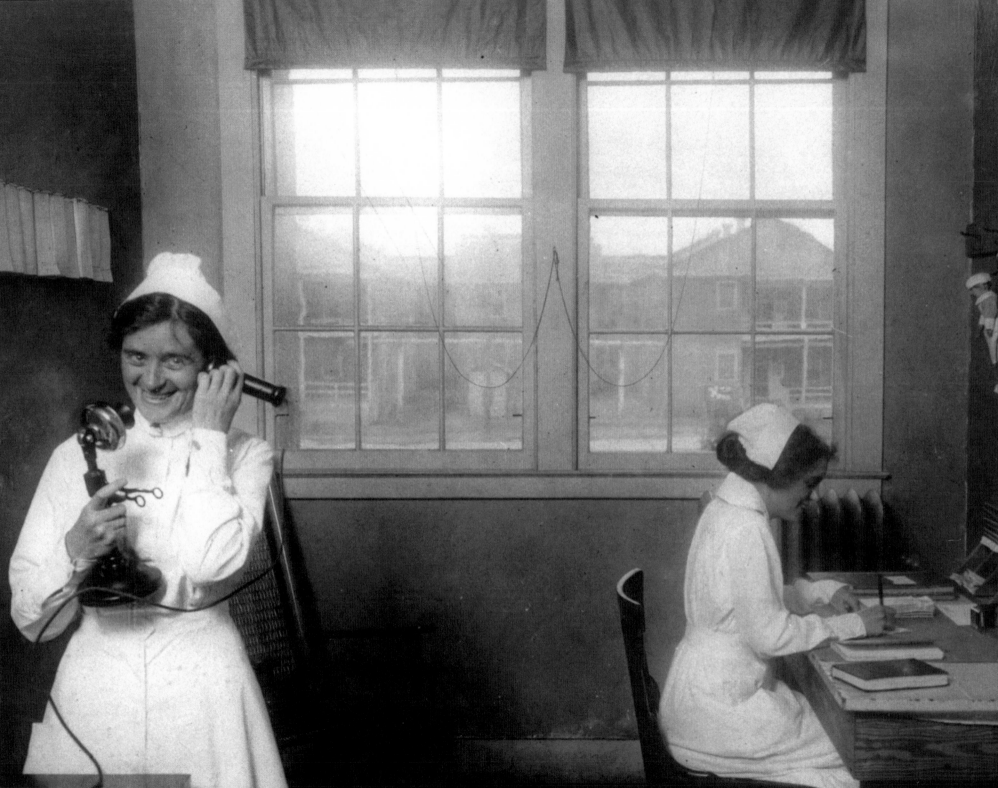

The Army Nurse Corps Goes Over there!

"IN 1910 NURSES' PAY WAS INCREASED TO $50 A MONTH, with $5 increase for every three years' completed service, for a period of nine years, making the maximum pay $65 a month after nine years' service. The act of July 9, 1918, increased the base pay to $60 per month and maintenance with $5 per month increase for each completed three years' service, and an additional $5 increase after 12 years' service. This act also provided for $30 per month additional pay for all chief nurses and $10 per month extra for foreign service.

"Army nurses who reported for duty on or before November 11, 1918, and whose service was honourable, were entitled to the $60 bonus upon their separation from the service.

"Both before and during the World War, nurses, although a part of the army, were considered as neither enlisted nor commissioned personnel." (*The Medical Dept in the World War, Vol. XIII, p. 300*)

Army nurses in Vera Cruz, Mexico, during the Punitive Expedition (March 1916–February 1917), wore gray crepe duty uniforms. While that uniform's original color was sensible and practical, the gray dresses were considered unbecoming and washed poorly, fading into a shapeless garment of myriad running colors. Jane Delano preferred the gray uniform, but The Surgeon General overrode her choice and directed that Army nurses wear a prescribed white dress.

Nurse Estelle Hines wearing the authorized white uniform.

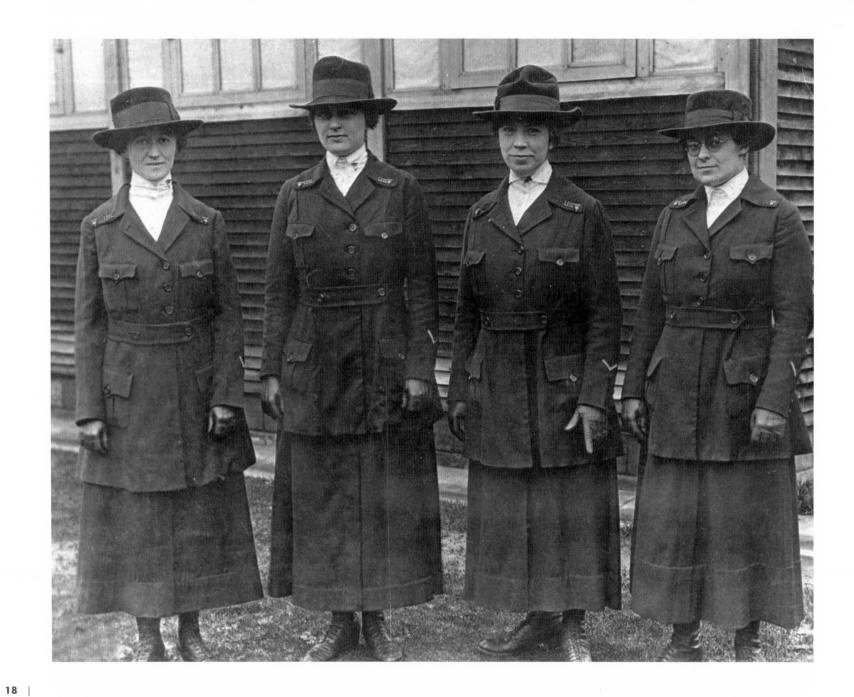

The uniform of September 1917 was adapted from that of 1899, with modifications made in 1910 and 1915. It consisted of a shirtwaist (blouse), skirt, belt, collar, cap, and the badge of the Corps, which was a gold caduceus superimposed in the center by the letters "A.N.C." in white enamel.

"Previous to the time that the United States entered the World War and particularly before members of the Army Nurse Corps were sent overseas, there was no prescribed outdoor uniform for the corps. When, however, nurses were ordered to Europe in the spring of 1917, the need for an outdoor uniform was appreciated, not only for reasons of convenience and economy but also for purposes of identification. Therefore, on May 17, 1917, the Surgeon General recommended to the War Department that an outdoor uniform for nurses, consisting of an olive-drab woollen skirt, coat and overcoat, a hat, a white or olive-drab shirt waist, and tan shoes be adopted. Since the suddenly increased demand for olive-drab materials would have made such a uniform most difficult to obtain, the plan to have this material was discarded, and on May 31, 1917, the blue-serge outdoor uniform of the Army Nurse Corps was adopted. Part of this outdoor uniform was a dark-blue serge Norfolk suit, with which either white or navy-blue shirt waists were to be worn. Besides this were the dark-blue overcoat, the hat, tan shoes, and tan gloves. The caduceus and the letters 'U.S.' in bronze were to be worn with this uniform, but on May 31, 1917, upon recommendation of the Surgeon General, the Secretary of War approved the change in the badge by the addition of the letters 'A.N.C.' superimposed on the caduceus in gilt. This uniform was to be worn at such times as the Surgeon General might prescribe, and might be worn at any other time when the nurse was not on duty." (*The Medical Dept in the World War, Vol. XIII, p. 302*)

"In August, 1917, legislation was proposed to provide members of the Army Nurse Corps with a suitable clothing allowance, but the Quartermaster General recommended as an alternative that an increase in pay be procured and that nurses be required to furnish their own uniforms. In consequence, the monthly pay of nurses was increased $10 only, which proved inadequate in view of the fact that the increase in cost of uniform equipment was proportionately greater. . . . Although the Army did increase nurses' monthly pay by ten dollars, this was insufficient to pay for the expense of outfitting nurses for wartime services. By default, the Red Cross continued to contribute to the nurses' clothing needs for the duration of the war. Only in 1922 did the government finally reimburse the Red Cross for all its uniform and equipment expenses." (*The Medical Dept in the World War, Vol. XIII, p. 303*)

(Opposite) *Nurses at Camp Hospital No. 29, Le Courneau, Gironde, France, 29 December 1918.*

"The regulation uniform is to be worn by nurses and reserve nurses of the Army Nurse Corps at all times, and is as follows:

"A suit, waist, and hat, of prescribed color and pattern for out door wear; gray or white uniforms, aprons and caps, will be worn while on duty in hospital, and shall be made in accordance with specifications furnished by the office of the Surgeon General, but reserve nurses will wear caps made in accordance with specifications furnished by the Red Cross; white, tan or black shoes, high or low, may be worn, but pumps, French heels and fancy shoes, will not be allowed; the U.S. pin and the insignia of the A.N.C. should be worn but not fancy pins or furs. There are no occasions when the wearing of civilian dress will be permitted, and any individual modification of the regulation uniform will not be allowed." (*Circular No. 30, 23 May 1918, M.W. Ireland, Brig Gen. M.C., U.S.A., Chief Surgeon*)

"For the thousands of new members of the Army, there was no indication upon the uniform to show to what class the nurses belonged, and on account of this in many cases they were not accorded the respect commensurate with the dignity and responsibility of their position. Such experiences during the war demonstrated that a different status and a recognition of it would have to be awarded Army nurses in order to interest future desirable nurses in the service and also to retain those already there, but the main argument for rank was the need of a definite status." (*The Medical Dept in the World War, Vol. XIII, p. 304*)

"Weather is much cooler, yesterday I dressed up in our new suit and went to church for a change. The suit looks like a Halsted St. bargain but it is better than what we have been wearing. We received new gray jersey dresses from the Red Cross. They look very well and will be warmer for the cold days ahead. I will wear mine now as the nights are cold. We were issued trench coats, rain proof, warm and very good looking. . . ." (*August 5, 1918, Maude Frances Essig, Reserve Army Nurse Corps*)

(Opposite) *For the first few months of the mobilization, the Red Cross provided the nurses with uniform apparel onboard ship just before sailing.*

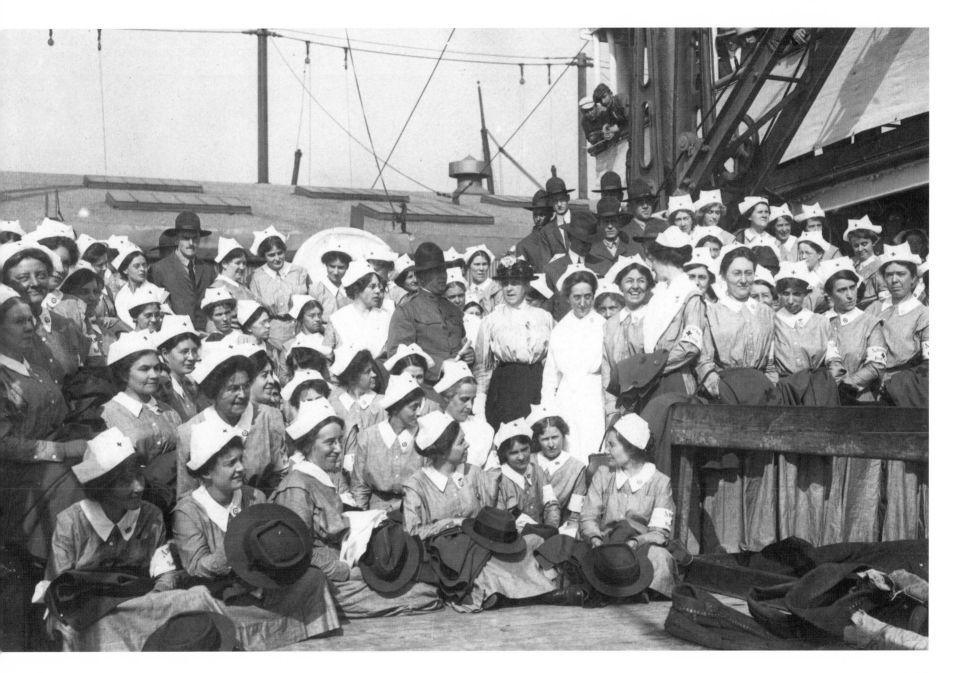

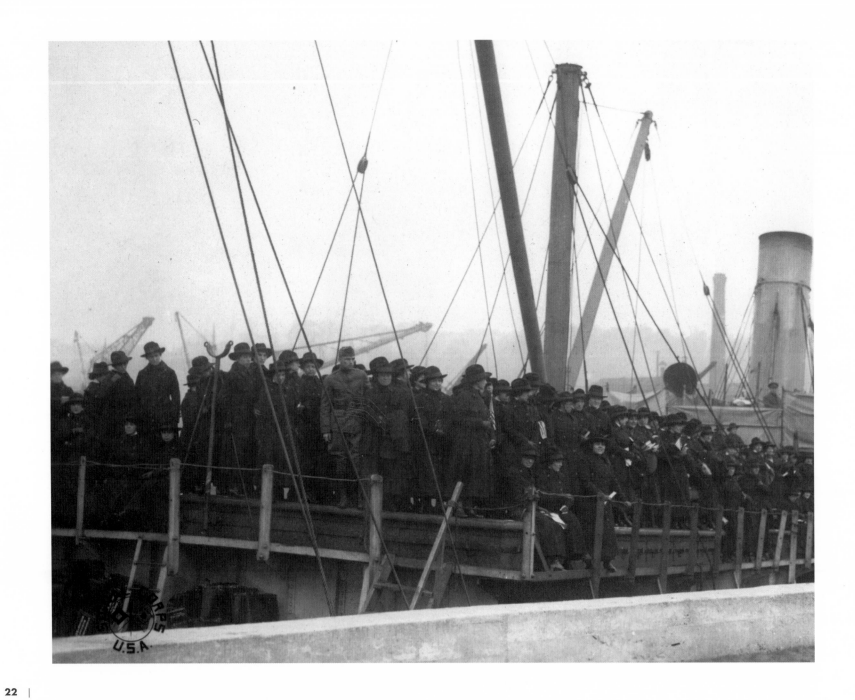

The first mobilization station for nurses was opened June 15, 1917, with its headquarters at the U.S. Quarantine Hospital, Ellis Island, New York. This station eventually accommodated approximately 350 nurses, but as the numbers awaiting mobilization for overseas duty increased, nurses were repeatedly shuffled from one site to another in the New York City/New Jersey area.

In the hospital units that went overseas before any nurses' mobilization stations existed, nurses usually accompanied the medical officers of their respective base hospitals, not knowing their destination. They received their orders within the shortest possible period of time before sailing, and received much less equipment than units that sailed later.

"Days spent at the mobilization stations were full of interest and intense excitement. Every morning each nurse had to be present at roll call, followed by military drill. After the matter of passports, inoculations, uniform, and equipment had been attended to, there were the rounds of shopping and sightseeing. It should be noted here, however, that nurses were never allowed to stay away from the mobilization station over night and only for a few hours at a time during the day, because it was never known when sailing orders for a unit might arrive." (*The Medical Dept in the World War, Vol. XIII, p. 308*)

"Difficulty was experienced in getting the nurses to understand how much baggage they could take overseas. In spite of instructions to the contrary, some would arrive at the point of mobilization with two or more trunks, several suit cases, and in many cases insufficient funds for their incidental needs. A memorandum was issued by the Surgeon General's Office early in January, 1918, which stated that nurses ordered abroad might take with them only a steamer trunk not exceeding 36 inches in length, one suit case or large satchel, and one blanket roll. It also advised each nurse to have if possible $50 in cash before leaving the United States." (*The Medical Dept in the World War, Vol. XIII, p. 308*)

"We are to move to another hotel tomorrow night. So the next letter you write send it to Old Colony Club, 120 Madison Ave., New York City. Don't know why we are going to move, after one has been in the army awhile you stop asking why, for you never know why this or that happens." *(July 12, 1918, Elizabeth Lewis, Evacuation Hospital No. 15, Hotel Arlington, New York)*

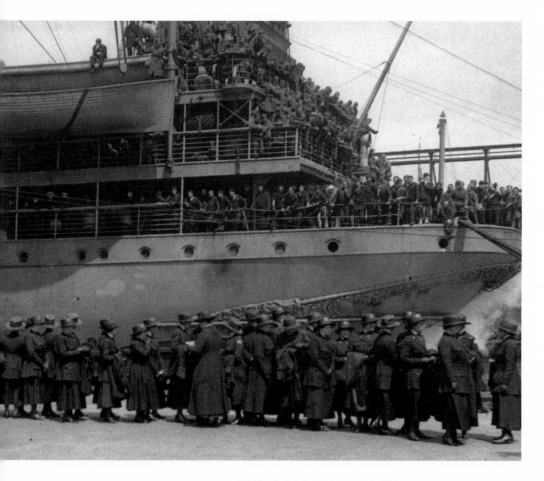

"We left St. Mary's and are now nicely deposited on Ellis Island. One step nearer 'over there'. I hope we go soon. I am very tired of my vacation—one can't manage on $10 a month so near the big City—this is a beautiful spot, the air is grand, and wonderful view of the Statue of Liberty. It is a view worth fighting for—place is closely guarded. 18 nurses to a ward—we lined up alphabetically and I have all new roommates. Good beds—a real treat after the buggy cots at St. Mary's[.] Good food, also in comparison. I feel satisfied for the first time since sojourning with Uncle Sam. Moonlight on the water and the Statue lit up made me sentimental. We have roll call at 9 and can have shore leave until midnight every day if we like. Go over on Gov't Ferry for free[;] Baggage received rough handling and I need a new bag." *(October 19, 1917, Maude Frances Essig)*

"Tuesday—we are still in dock. Weather fair, not cold. Good night considering our crowded quarters and the lack of Ellis Island's fresh air. One of the crew fell into an open hatch last night and was killed. One negroe [sic] died of fright. Meals good but cold, at 7:30, 12 and 5. Roll call at 10:30 and 3:30. Ship abandon drill at 2:00. Walked deck and played 500 to pass away the time. Retired early, not allowed on deck when we pull out, so no use to sit up. We sailed at 11 PM." *(December 4, 1917, Maude Frances Essig)*

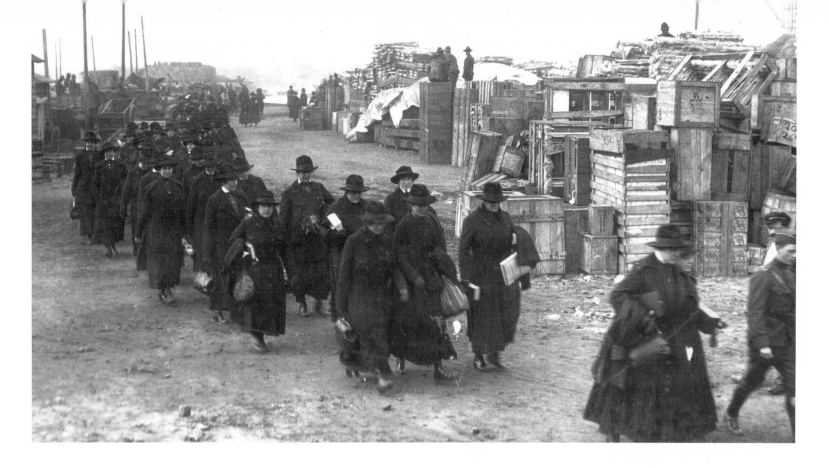

"Thursday—land was sighted at 11:00 AM. Wonderful! First in view was a lighthouse, then several rocky mounds came into view. In one half hour, we could dimly see the outline of the rugged coastline of Brittany, slowly coast defenses, wireless stations and more lighthouses came into sight as we entered the Bay of Brest.

"We anchored close to the bank breakwater, where we are to stay for a time. We mailed our letters with someone going a shore. Everybody very happy once more." (*December 20, 1917, Maude Frances Essig*)

"Monday—fair and warmer. We left the big gray boat by launch about 9 AM. We stood in line for ages waiting our turn to walk up a high bluff. We arrived at R.R. Station, Brest, France, at 10:00. Everything beautifully green and all is so strange. Truly a foreign land. Saw only a few Americans." (*December 24, 1917, Maude Frances Essig*)

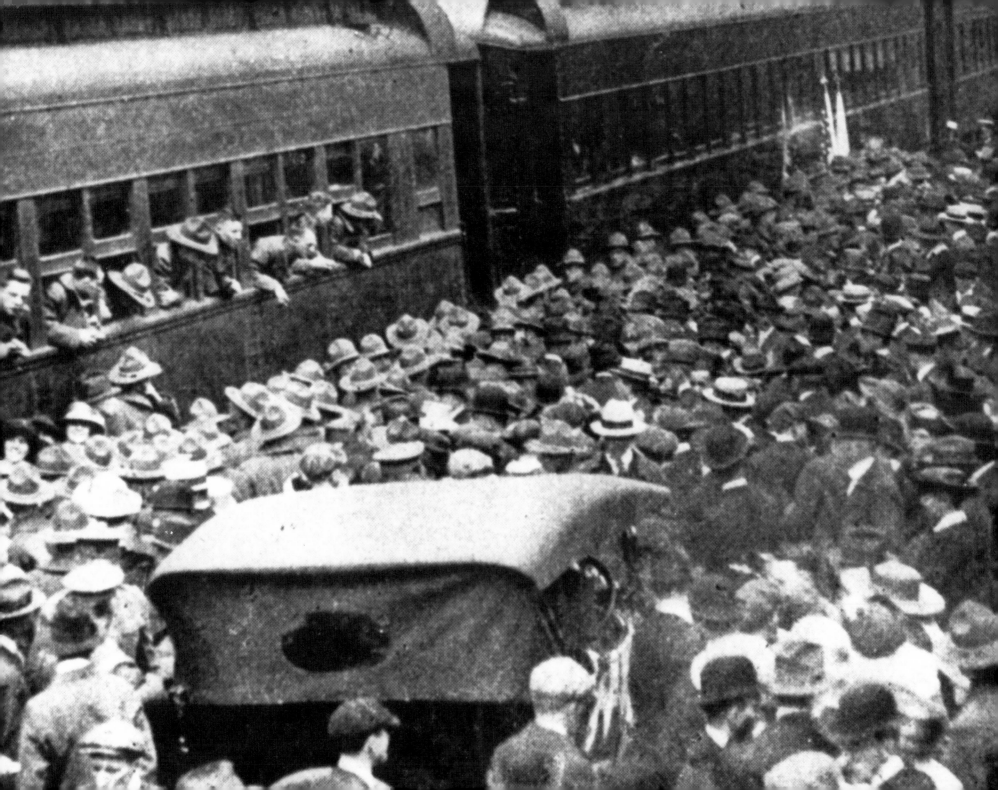

The Army Medical Department and the Red Cross

WHEN WORLD WAR I BROKE OVER EUROPE IN AUGUST 1914, the American Red Cross offered its trained personnel and hospital supplies to every belligerent country. On September 13, 1914, the relief ship *Red Cross* carried surgeons, supplies, and 120 nurses to England, Russia, France, Germany, Austria, Belgium, Serbia, and Bulgaria. Most units returned to America in October 1915, but some members remained as volunteers. Red Cross nurses were still serving in all of the Allied countries when the American forces arrived.

The experience of the Red Cross nurses serving overseas proved invaluable when the United States entered the war and the nurses were mobilized for immediate action. The Red Cross mobilized 2,970 of the 8,015 names on their list of volunteers, enough to care for an army of a million men, according to the calculations of the day.

A year before the United States entered war, The Surgeon General had requested that the Red Cross organize base hospital units. These base hospitals became the hospital system that served as the backbone of the Medical Department during the first trying months of the war. The largest civilian hospitals and medical schools of America were called on to organize teams from their staffs, with doctors and nurses accustomed to working together, and soon a score of units known as "affiliates" were established. Twenty-two doctors, two dentists, sixty-five Red Cross nurses, one hundred and fifty-three enlisted men, six civilian employees, and a chaplain completed the personnel roster for a base hospital unit. Each member pledged to report for duty whenever called within two years.

The names of the affiliate nurses were submitted to the Bureau of Nursing Service at Red Cross Headquarters and held for final assignment to the Army Nurse Corps. The volunteers then scattered to their daily jobs and civilian lives until they received the call to duty, which could require their presence at very short notice.

Red Cross Hospitals

"THESE HOSPITALS WERE PERMITTED TO FUNCTION in the zone of the armies only through urgent necessity. The Medical Department was at all times so short of material that it became necessary in emergencies to call upon the Red Cross to furnish tentage, equipment, and some personnel to meet our needs. These hospitals functioned in the same manner as our own evacuation hospitals and under the command of an officer of the medical Department. They rendered exceptionally efficient service. Two of them were utilized during the Chateau-Thierry operations, and two during the St. Mihiel-Argonne offensives." (*Annual Report of the Surgeon General U.S. Army to the Secretary of War, 1919, Vol. II, Washington Government Printing Office, 1919 [hereafter Surgeon General Report, 1919], Vol. II, p. 1467*)

Once America entered the war with Germany, 25 base hospital units were well under way. The first call for specific aid came to America through the British Commission for doctors and nurses. Six of the waiting base hospital units were assigned to duty with the British Expeditionary Force. Base Hospital No. 4 was the first to leave New York in May 1917; No. 5 followed two days later; and then Nos. 2, 12, 21 and 10. The first American flag to fly in alliance over France was at the hospital unit in Rouen.

In the first seven months after America joined the war, 17 base hospital units were rushed to France, and the others were held in readiness for immediate departure. The base hospitals and their personnel, organized and equipped by the Red Cross, automatically became part of the Army organization when they were sent into service overseas.

"Early in August 1918, all the base hospitals organized by the American Red Cross nursing service, Nos. 1 to 50, had been sent to Europe. Base Hospitals No. 51 upward to No. 79, and the special hospitals, No. 102 for duty in Italy, No. 114 for orthopedic cases, No. 115 for head surgery, No. 116 for fracture cases, and No. 117 for psychiatric cases were organized in the Army Nurse Corps division of the Surgeon General's Office. The personnel was selected from among those nurses who had proved themselves professionally and physically fit for duty in the cantonments [in the U.S.]. There were 1,445 nurses at the port of embarkation awaiting sailing orders, en route to the mobilization station, or under orders to mobilize when the armistice was signed. Of the number awaiting sailing orders 650 were sent overseas upon the request of the chief surgeon American Expeditionary Forces." (*Surgeon General Report, 1919, Vol. II, p. 1123*)

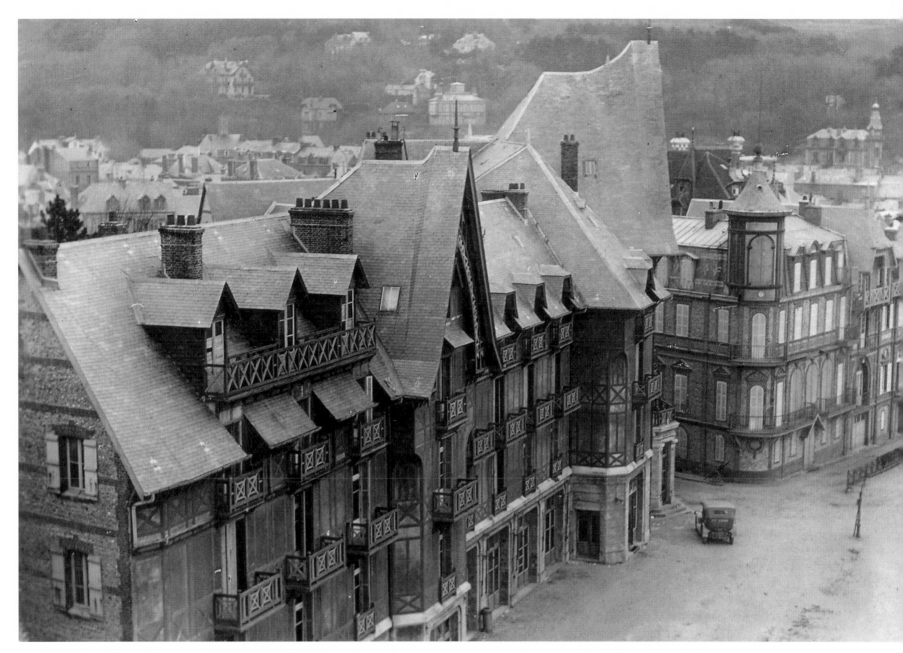

Base Hospital No. 2, Etretat, France.

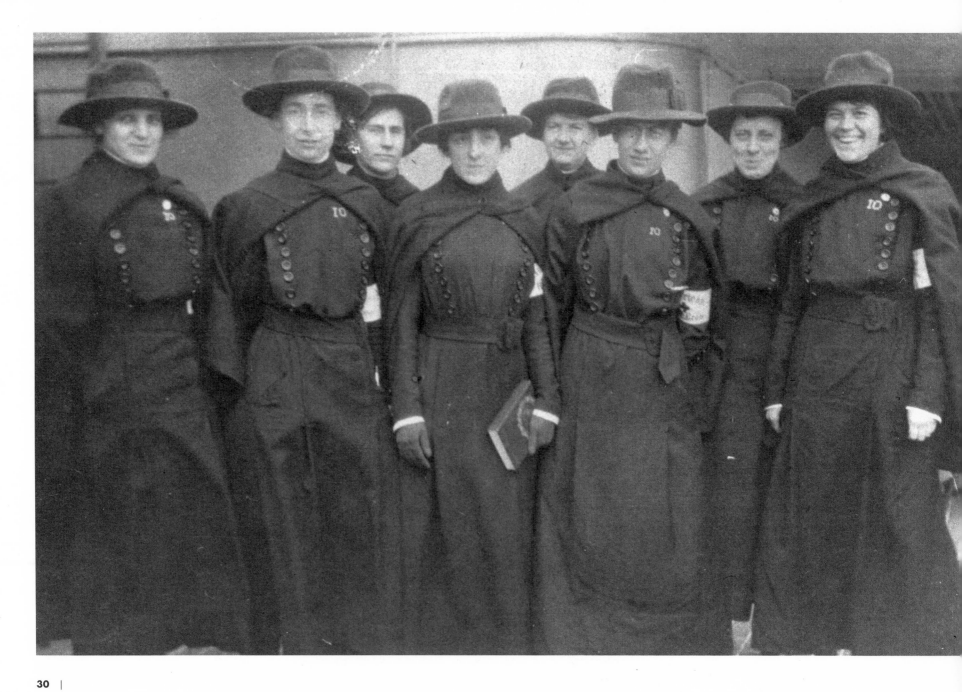

Within six months after the United States entered the war, approximately 1,100 nurses had sailed overseas, about half of whom were stationed with their base hospital units in six British general hospitals. The first base hospital units to sail took over British facilities as follows, shortly after their arrival in France:

- **Base Hospital No. 4** (Lakeside Hospital Unit, Cleveland, Ohio) sailed May 7, 1917, and took over No. 9 British General Hospital, Rouen, France.

- **Base Hospital No. 5** (Harvard University, Boston, Mass.) sailed May 11, 1917, and took over No. 11 British General Hospital and later No. 13 British General Hospital, Bologne, France.

- **Base Hospital No. 2** (Presbyterian Hospital Unit, New York, NY) sailed May 12, 1917, and took over No. 1 British General Hospital, Etretat, France.

- **Base Hospital No. 21** (Washington University Medical School Unit, St. Louis, Mo.), sailed May 19, 1917, and took over No. 12 British General Hospital, Rouen, France.

- **Base Hospital No. 10** (Pennsylvania Hospital Unit, Philadelphia, Pa.), sailed May 19, 1917, and took over No. 16 British General Hospital, Le Treport, France.

- **Base Hospital No. 12** (Northwestern University Medical School Unit, Chicago, Ill.) sailed May 24, 1917, and took over No. 18 British General Hospital, Dannes-Camiers, France.

"The hospitals taken over by the American units had been functioning actively for three years, and from the beginning of that period had seldom less than 900 or 1,000 patients, and very frequently more than that number in each. The British authorities made arrangements for each of the units to be met and conducted to the hospital which it was to take over. The British matron and a few of the nursing staff . . . remained for a certain length of time to assist the American staff in becoming acquainted with the ways of British hospitals." (*The Medical Dept in the World War, Vol. XIII, p. 317*)

(Opposite) *Nurses at Base Hospital No. 2, Etretat, France.*

Nurses at Base Hospital No. 2 in Etretat, France, out for a stroll around the town.

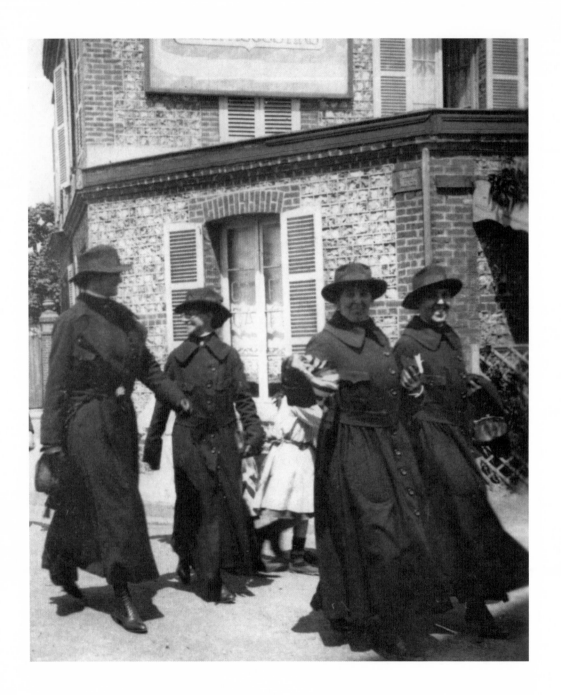

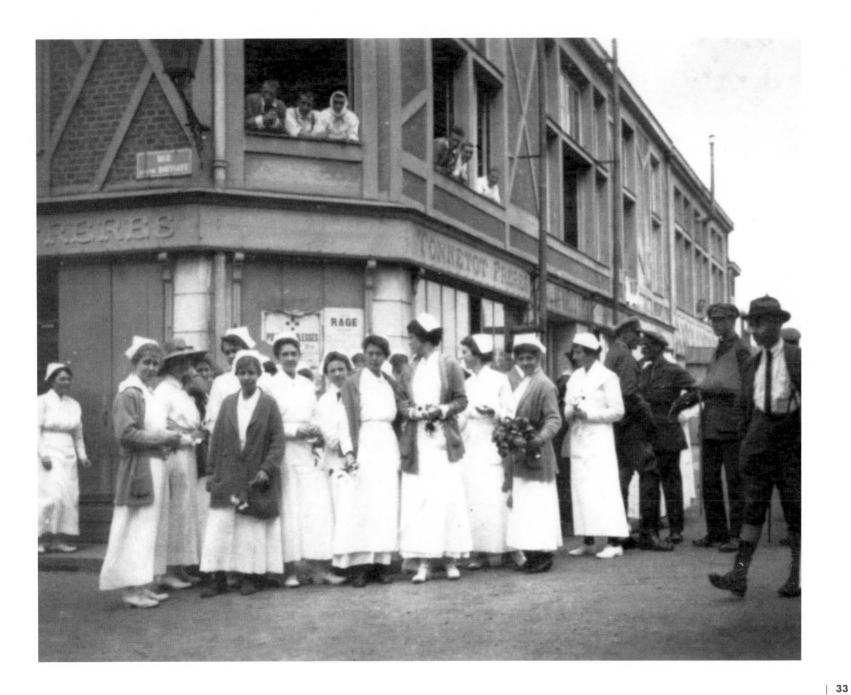

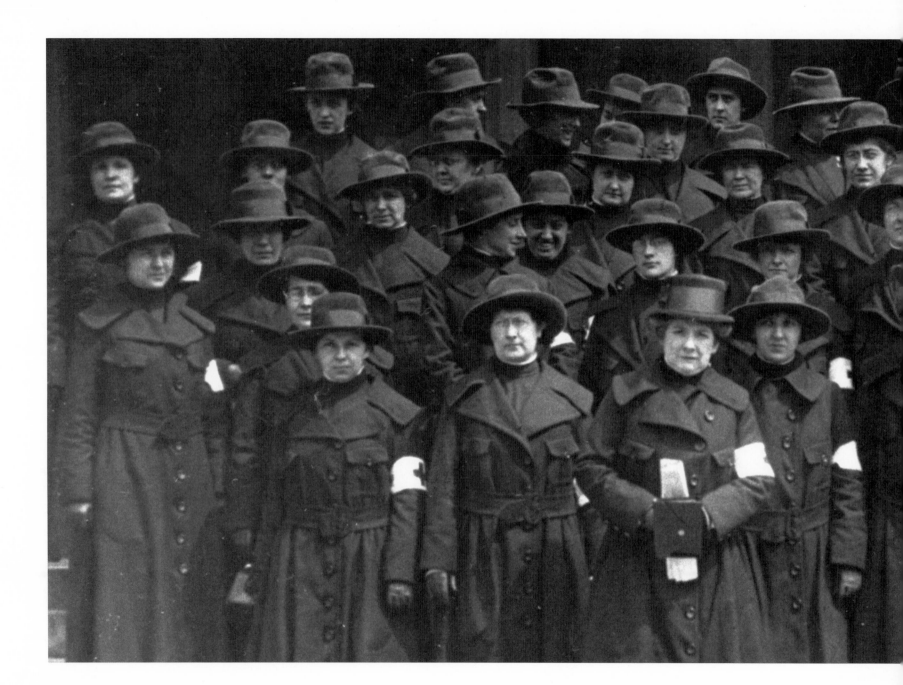

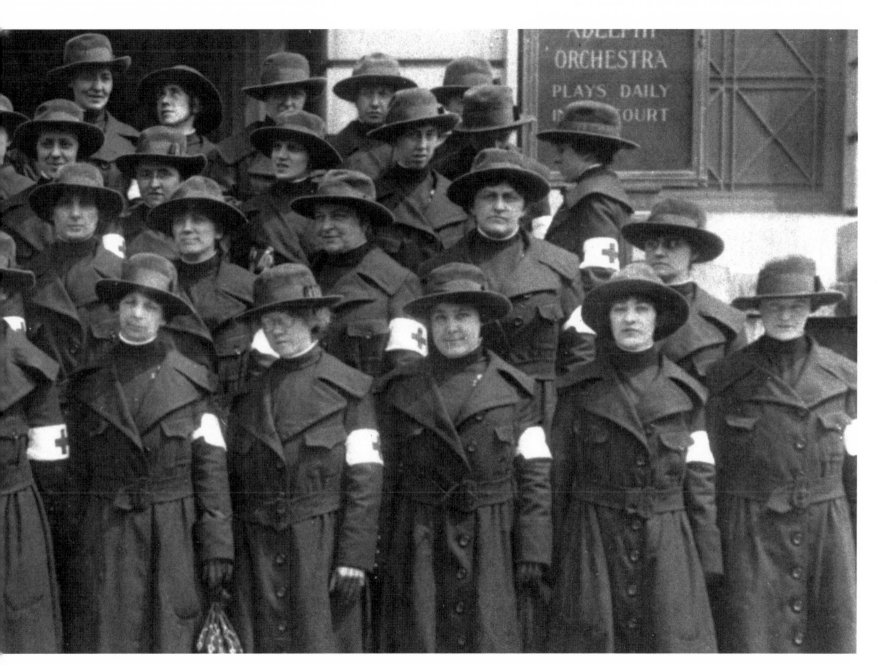

Nurses of Base Hospital No.10 in Liverpool, England, on their way to France, May 1917.

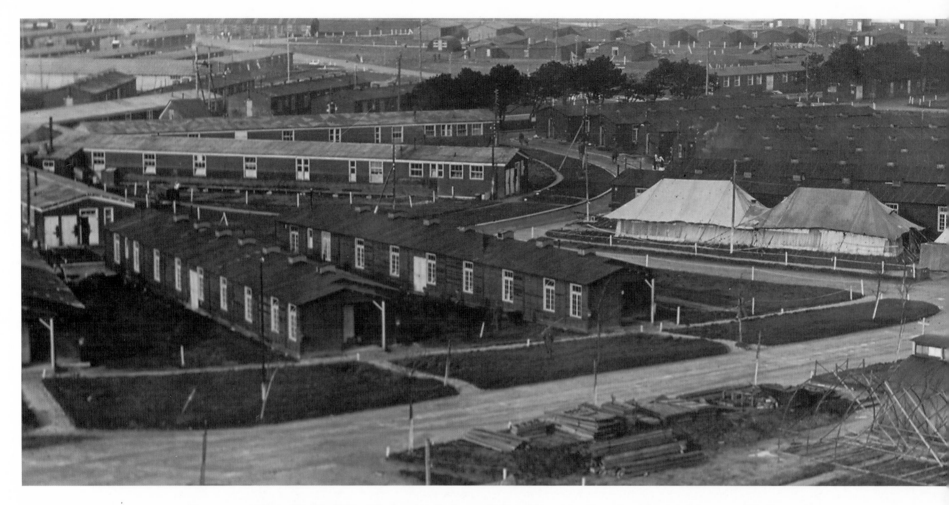

Panorama of Base Hospital No. 10, showing the latest design of location of wards and operating room. The latter is in the center of the circle. Le Treport, Seine-Infereiure, France.

British General Hospital No. 16 in the French fishing village of Le Treport had a bed capacity of 2,232 and was constructed entirely of huts. Upon arrival, Base Hospital No. 10 received 1,400 patients during its first week of operations, mostly surgical and mustard gas cases.

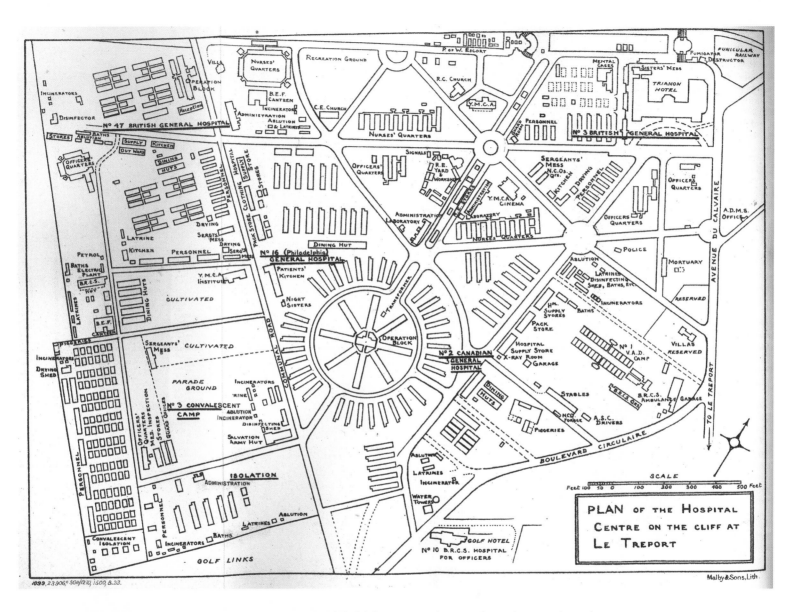

Plan of Base Hospital No. 10, at Le Treport. Note No. 16 (Philadelphia) General Hospital may be seen above the *"Operation Block."* (History of the Great War: Medical Services General History, Vol. II)

"Miss [Margaret] Dunlop, the Directress of Nurses at the Pennsylvania Hospital, was unanimously selected to be in charge of the nursing department. By this selection the Unit was most fortunate, as Miss Dunlop relied not only upon her own civil experience, but had the additional military and war experience gained while she was in charge of the American Ambulance at Neuilly, France." *(Pennsylvania Hospital Unit in the Great War)*

As chief nurse of Base Hospital No. 10, Miss Dunlop wore the mandatory half-inch black band on each sleeve of her outdoor uniform. She also has two service stripes on her sleeve representing her two years overseas.

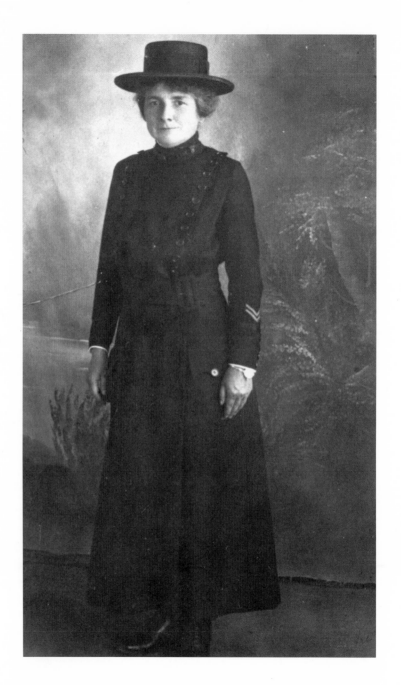

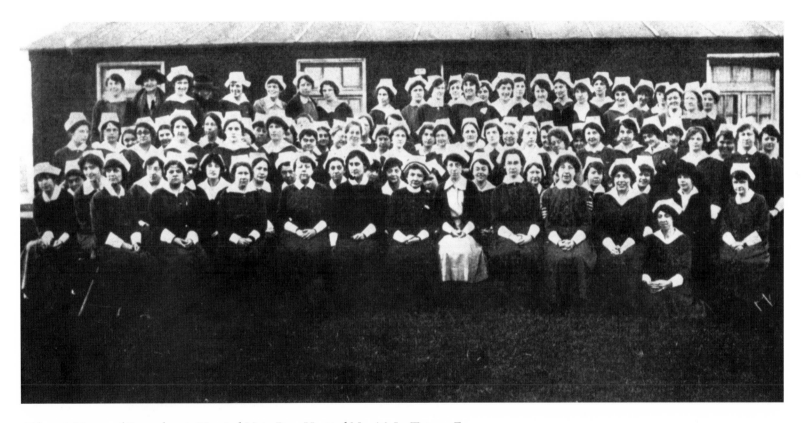

(Above) *Nurses of Pennsylvania Hospital Unit, Base Hospital No. 16, Le Treport, France.*

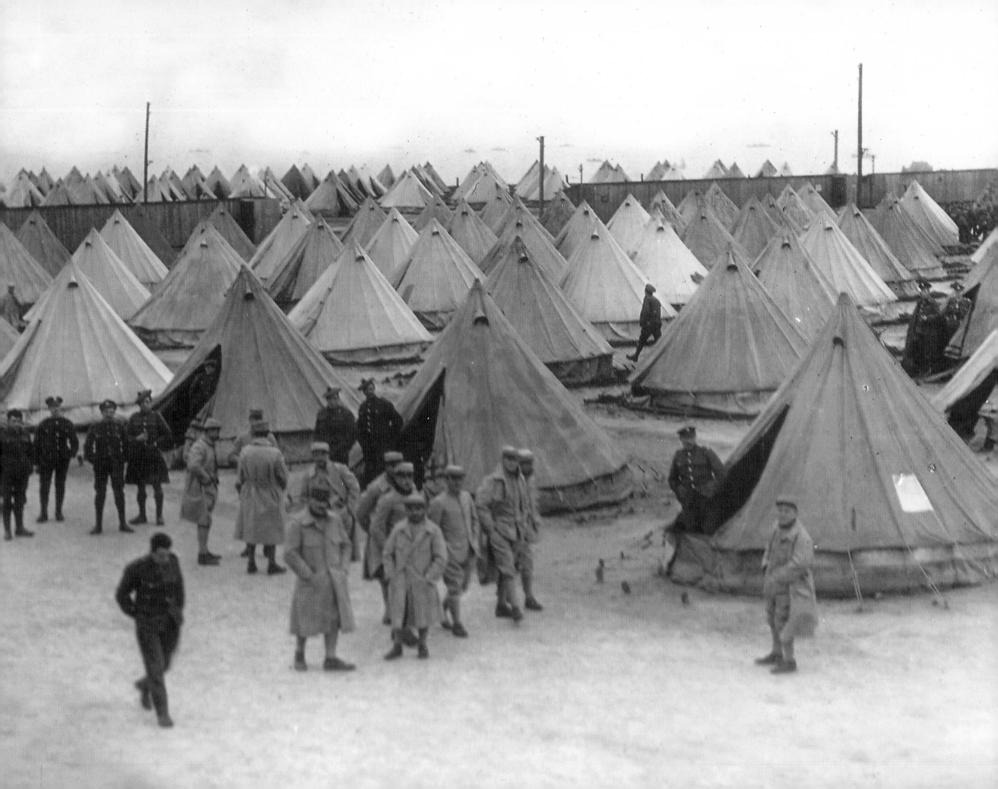

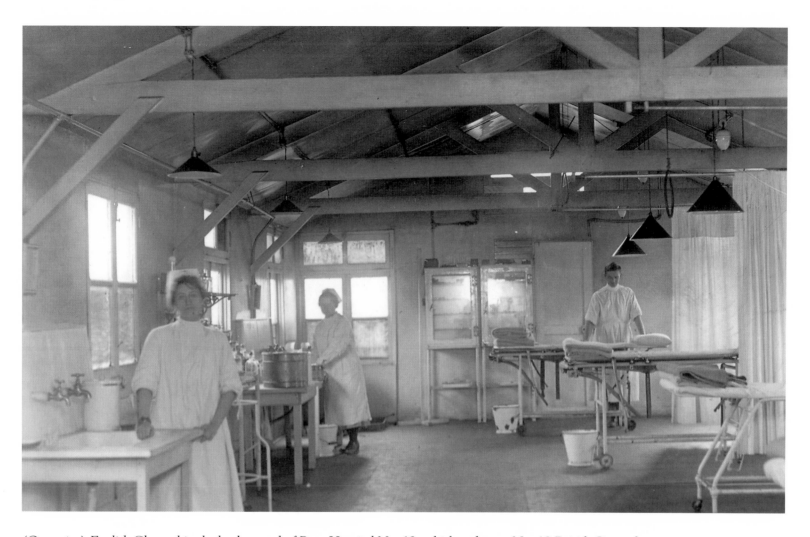

(Opposite) *English Channel in the background of Base Hospital No. 12, which took over No. 18 British General Hospital, Dannes-Camiers (Calais, France), December 17, 1918. When the unit sailed on the SS Mongolia, the ship's guns misfired and shell fragments hit and killed two nurses and wounded a third.*

(Above) *Operating room of the "larger" type. Taken at American Base Hospital No. 12, British Base Hospital No. 18, Dannes-Camiers, Pas-de-Calais, France, December 18, 1918.*

When the first call for U.S. medical aid came from overseas in 1917, dozens of U.S. doctors were dispatched to serve as medical officers with British infantry units at the front, and six of the waiting base hospitals were assigned to duty with the British Expeditionary Force. Among these was Base Hospital No. 21, organized by Washington University Medical School in St. Louis, Missouri. This unit was sent to Rouen, France, with Julia C. Stimson as chief nurse. *(Gavin I, p. 46)*

As Stimson wrote home from Rouen in March 1918, "patients began to pour in upon us. . . . Day before yesterday we operated on 50 cases, yesterday 51, today they had 73 scheduled. . . . They have at least 40 more cases to operate on tonight. . . . More convoys are due tonight. The doctors are about dead. They are working in shifts as much as they can. The stretcher-bearers are dead tired, but as cheerful as monkeys." *(Gavin quoting Stimson, American Women in WW1, p. 47)*

(Opposite) Red Cross nurses (prior to receiving Army Nurse Corps uniforms) getting water in front of their kitchen at Base Hospital No. 21, formerly stables for a race track. To one side, in front is Mense Taylor, chief nurse (in gray uniform). Rouen, Seine Inferieur, France.

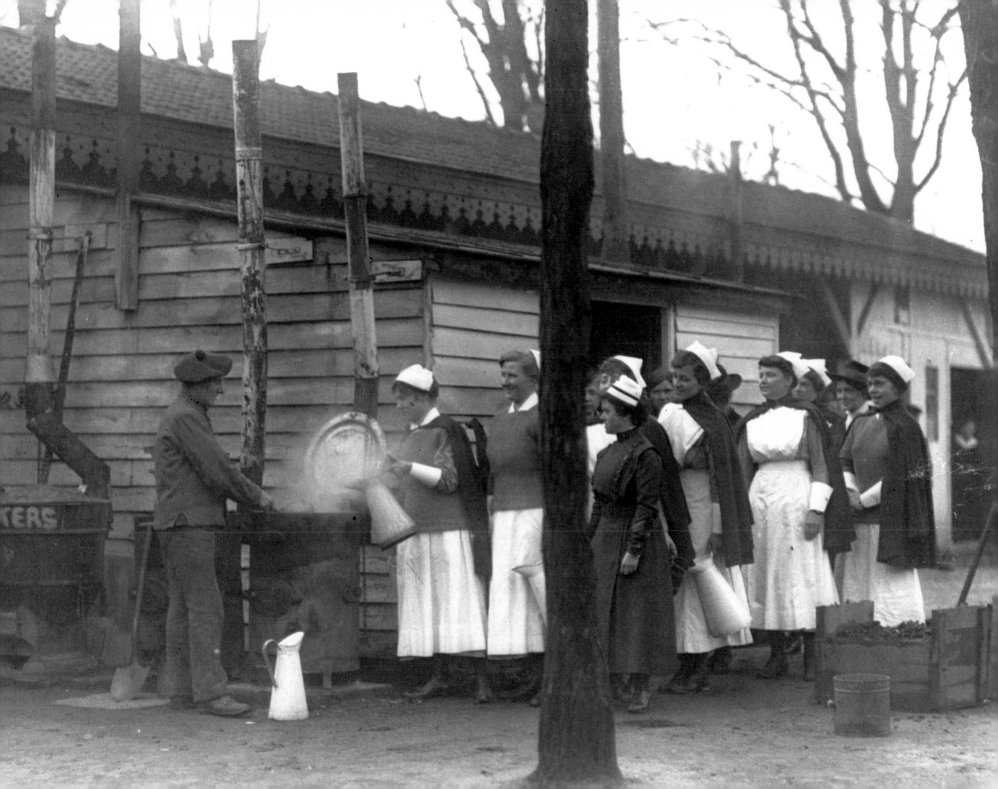

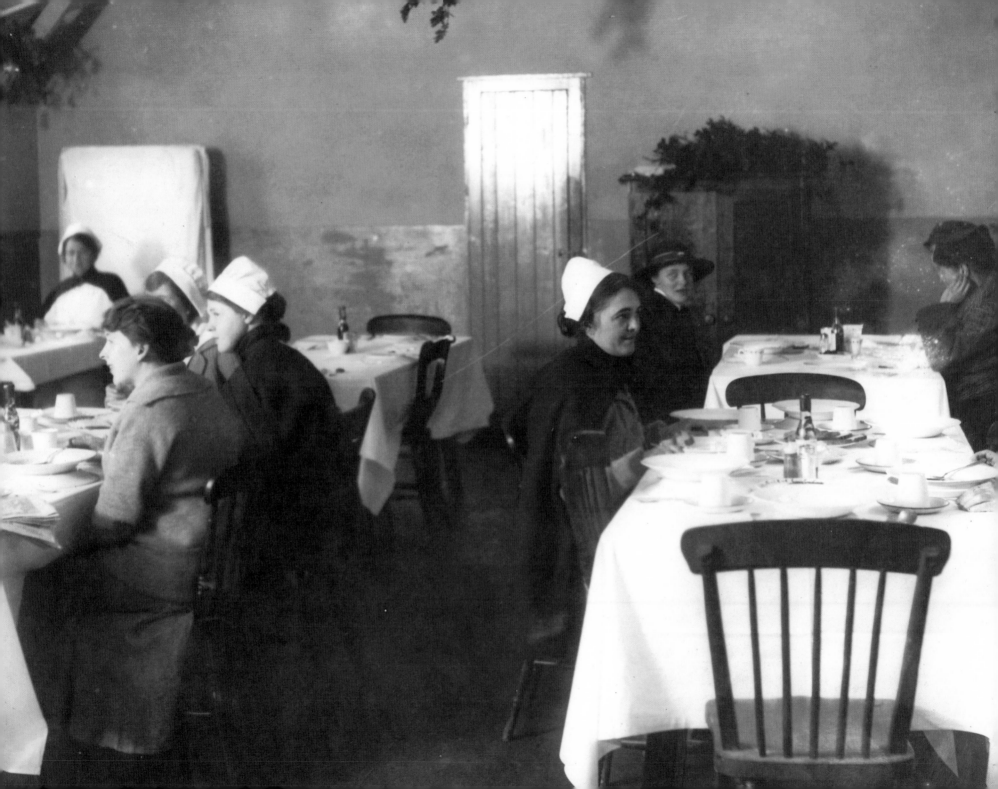

The Army Nurse in England

"IN JUNE, 1918, AN ARMY CHIEF NURSE and an assistant were assigned to duty in the office of the chief surgeon of Base Section No. 3, England. These two executives relieved two nurses who had been on duty in that office since the February preceding. Their duties consisted of the general supervision of all the nursing personnel of United States hospitals in Great Britain."

"Ten hospitals with American Army nurses functioned in this section, and three of these were American Red Cross military hospitals. During the influenza epidemic of October, 1918, 300 nurses en route to France were attached temporarily to the hospitals in this section where they were most vitally needed." *(The Medical Dept in the World War, Vol. XIII, p. 345)*

"During the war period 24 American-trained nurses, the majority of whom were British subjects, were transferred from the American Red Cross nursing service to the Army Nurse Corps while they were on duty in Base Section No. 3." *(The Medical Dept in the World War, Vol. XIII, p. 345)*

(Opposite) *Nurses' dining room, Winchester, England.*

(Right) *American Red Cross nurses' club operated in connection with the American soldiers' camp hospital at Romsey, England.*

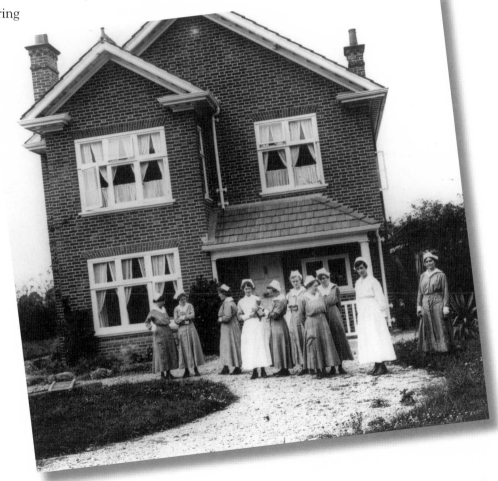

Stateside Nursing

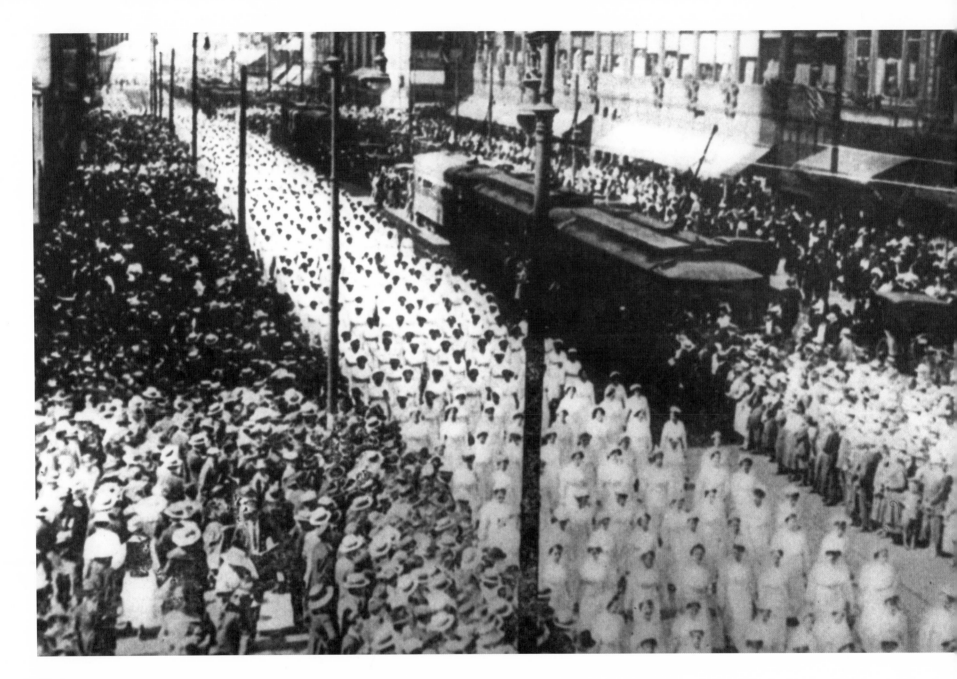

The Army School of Nursing

UPON THE RECOMMENDATION OF THE SURGEON GENERAL of the Army, Secretary of War Newton Baker approved the establishment of the Army School of Nursing on May 25, 1918, during the height of World War I.

As soon as the plan was accepted, the Women's Committee of the Council of National Defense, the Red Cross, and the Nursing Committee of the General Medical Board, plunged into a recruiting campaign. Within five months of the school's establishment, 11,000 applications were filed. Between July 24, 1918, and February of the following year, the school offered courses of instruction at 31 U.S. base hospitals.

The Army School of Nursing was unique and highly respected. By the time of the armistice in November 1918, the school had accepted 5,267 of the 10,689 women who applied for admission. During its entire existence, from 1918 until 1933, the school graduated 937 trained nurses, 28% of whom joined the Army Nurse Corps. *(Sarnecky, pp. 86–87)*

Annie Warburton Goodrich (1866–1954), the first Dean of the Army School of Nursing, was born in New Brunswick, New Jersey, in 1866. She graduated from New Hospital School of Nursing in 1892, and served as superintendent of nursing at New York Post-Graduate Hospital, at St. Luke's Hospital, and at New York Hospital. In 1914 she was appointed assistant professor of nursing and health at Teachers College, Columbia University. In 1918 she became Dean of the Army School of Nursing, a position she held for 18 months.

Thanks to Goodrich's efforts, the sole use of trained graduate nurses overseas, rather than trained aides, became a matter of formal policy during World War I.

(Opposite) *Army and Navy nurses marching for recruitment on State Street, Chicago, Illinois, 1918.*

"During World War I, 21,480 women served as Army nurses. Most volunteered to go to France but only 10,245 or slightly less than half, realized their ambition. The others . . . did not serve with units on the field of combat. Many of the remainder served in the post hospitals, the cantonment hospitals, the general hospitals, hospitals at the coast artillery posts, the ports of embarkation and debarkation, the aviation stations, the arsenals and the recruit camps, on the hospital trains, in the nurses' mobilization stations, and in the surgeon generals' office within the United States. In short, they were the vital infrastructure of military nursing in the Zone of the Interior." *(Sarnecky, p. 122)*

The hospital structure in the continental United States burgeoned enormously to support the vastly expanded Army. By November 1918, the Medical Department managed 92 large hospitals (89 of them newly built) with 120,916 beds.

"Early in 1917, builders hastily erected cantonment or base hospitals according to a standard plan at the mobilization camps where the Army processed [and trained] masses of recruits. Most cantonment hospitals were one thousand-bed pavilion hospitals with corridors connecting the far flung buildings. Each building houses open wards for fourteen to one hundred patients with a private room near the nurses' station for those patients who required closer supervision." *(Sarnecky, p. 123)*

"A typical day in a cantonment hospital included certain set routines. At 0700 hours, nurses took patients' vital signs, bathed them, got convalescent patients out of bed, changed dressings, and gave necessary treatments. Then they prepared for the ward officer's 0900 inspection. Ward staff straightened beds and cleaned floors, utility rooms, latrines, diet kitchens, and refrigerators. Additionally, they collected and counted soiled linen, swept, dusted, mopped, and tended stoves by shovelling coal and removing ashes. After officers completed their rigid morning inspection, the staff provided nourishments. After dinner, those still seriously ill rested, the convalescent patients found some recreations, visitors came, and the nurses did their paperwork." *(Sarnecky, pp. 123–124)*

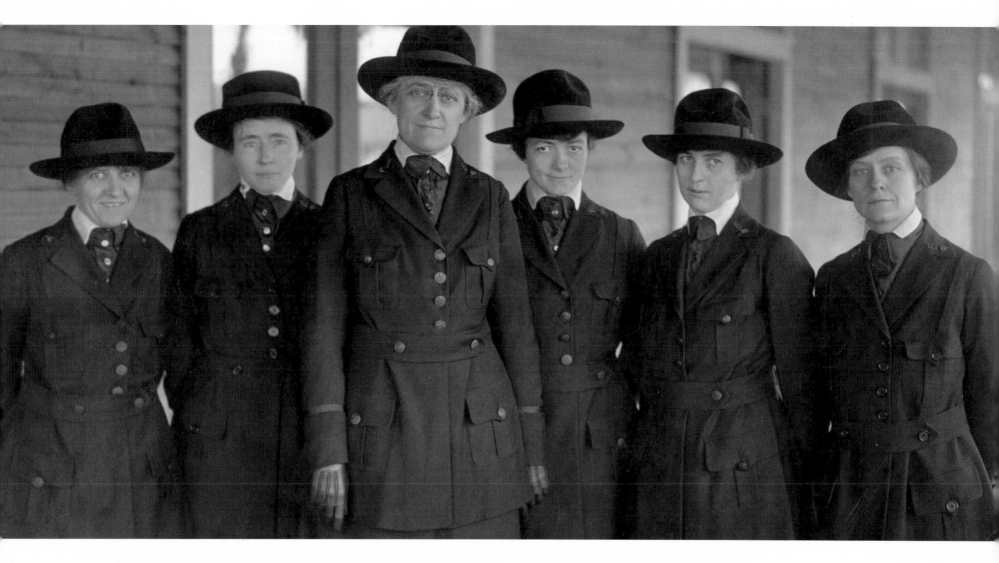

"Bill Bessie with unidentified nurses wearing blue velour hats." Bessie was formerly chief nurse at Walter Reed General Hospital. These nurses are at Eberts Field, Arkansas, which ranked second among aviation training fields maintained by the U.S. Government. About 1,500 enlisted men and officers were stationed at the field. (Note the half-inch black band on each sleeve of the outdoor uniform designating chief nurse status.)

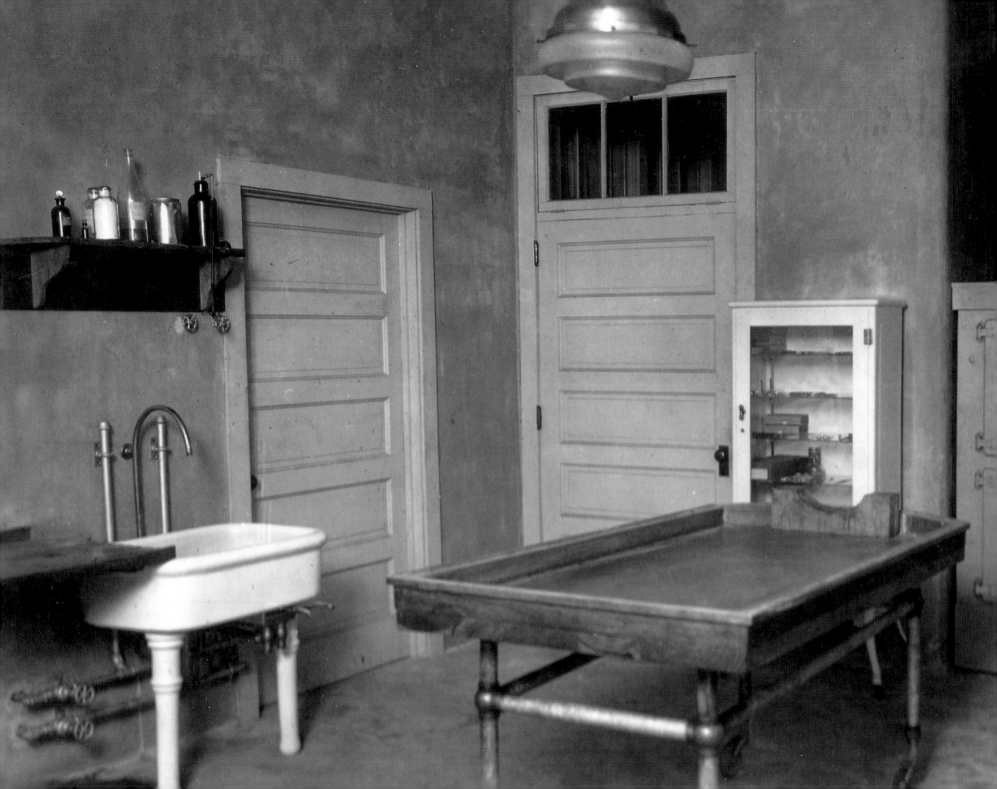

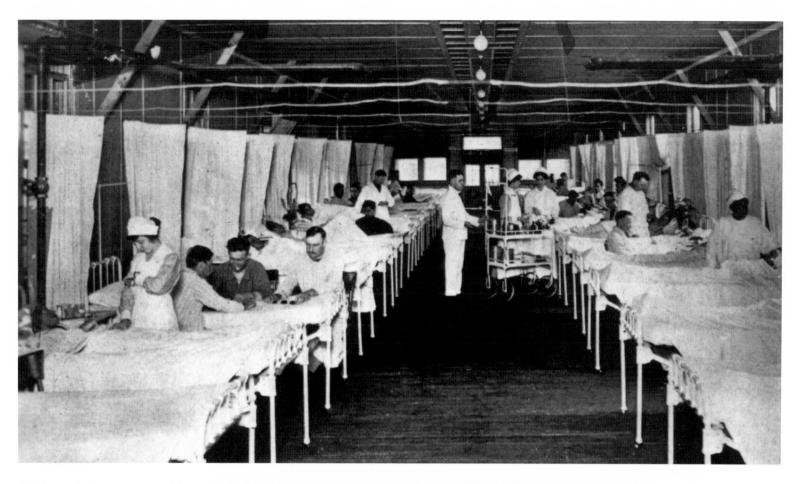

(Opposite) *Autopsy room, laboratory building, Base Hospital, Camp Mills, Long Island, NY. Camp Mills was situated near Mineola, Long Island, and because it was a tent camp, it was unusable during the winter of 1917–1918. During 1918 construction was started to provide barrack space for 50,000 troops.*

(Above) *"My boys not very sick. Have a great time with them. 62 patients admitted. Mostly measles. 750 pts in hospital, 5 more nurses arrived. Storms awfully hard and very cold. Went to town. Froze my ears and got back at 2 PM. Never again. Not much sleep. Got a coat and muff from Ma."* (JANUARY 11, 1918, JOCOBINA R. RIECKE, CAMP GRANT, ILL.)

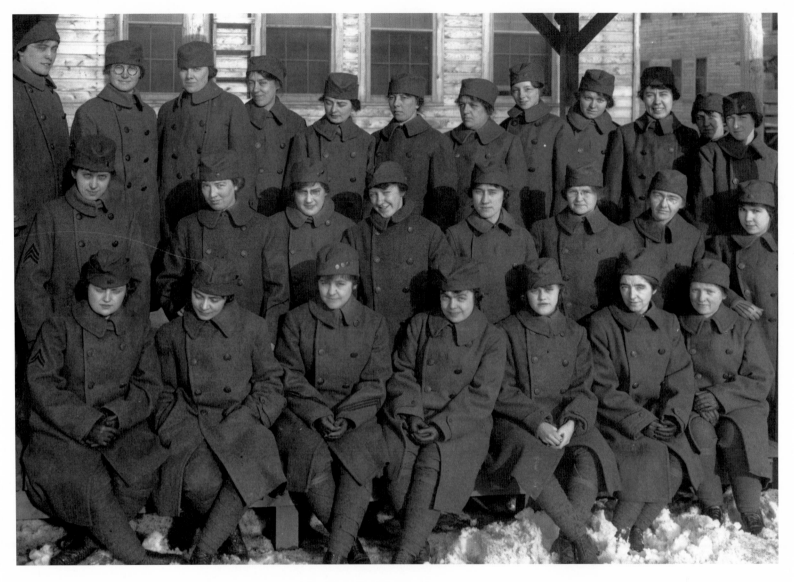

Nursing students from Company B, Camp Grant, Illinois, 1918. Cantonment hospitals in the north had heating plants but those in the south had no means of warmth; both staff and patients suffered from the intensely cold weather during the winter of 1917–1918.

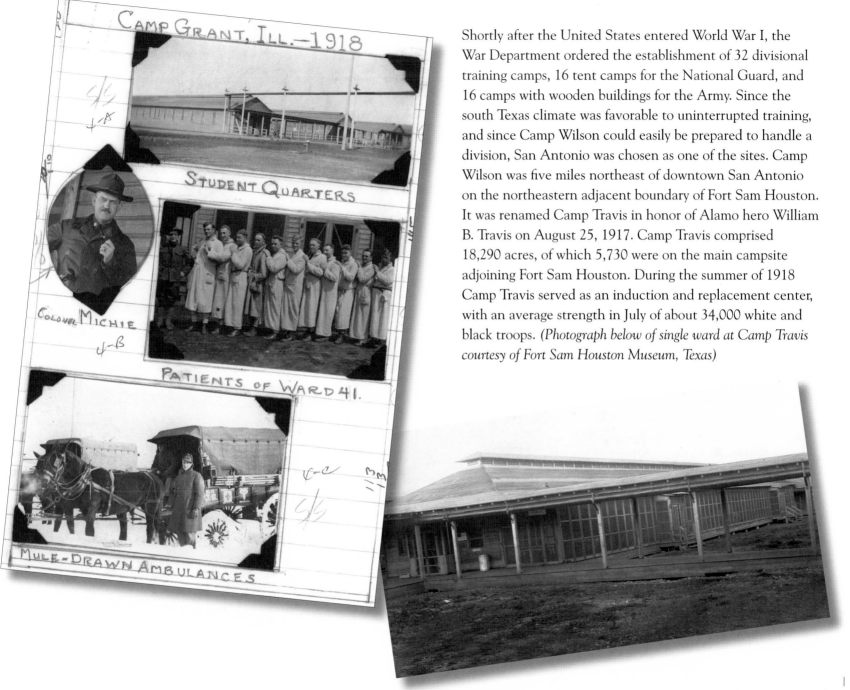

CAMP GRANT, ILL.—1918

STUDENT QUARTERS

COLONEL MICHIE

PATIENTS OF WARD 41.

MULE-DRAWN AMBULANCES

Shortly after the United States entered World War I, the War Department ordered the establishment of 32 divisional training camps, 16 tent camps for the National Guard, and 16 camps with wooden buildings for the Army. Since the south Texas climate was favorable to uninterrupted training, and since Camp Wilson could easily be prepared to handle a division, San Antonio was chosen as one of the sites. Camp Wilson was five miles northeast of downtown San Antonio on the northeastern adjacent boundary of Fort Sam Houston. It was renamed Camp Travis in honor of Alamo hero William B. Travis on August 25, 1917. Camp Travis comprised 18,290 acres, of which 5,730 were on the main campsite adjoining Fort Sam Houston. During the summer of 1918 Camp Travis served as an induction and replacement center, with an average strength in July of about 34,000 white and black troops. *(Photograph below of single ward at Camp Travis courtesy of Fort Sam Houston Museum, Texas)*

"The vast number of communicable diseases present in the fall of 1917 and the following winter prevented any great activity among the orthopaedic surgeons [at Camp Travis] until about February, 1918. The division surgeon . . . had obtained the incorporation of three excellent foot exercises in the prescribed setting-up exercises [for new recruits]. The three orthopaedists were assigned to the work of foot measurement and shoe fitting, in addition to their other duties, without being given any enlisted assistants. This resulted in the neglect of their other work, in the unsuccessful attempt to avoid interference with the progress of military training, until the work was reorganized by the division surgeon. Company supply sergeants were required to issue shoes of the sizes called for by actual foot measurements." (*The Medical Dept in the World War, Vol. IV, p. 139*)

(Left) *The book cart at Camp Travis, Texas.*

(Opposite) *The orthopedic ward at Camp Travis, Texas.*

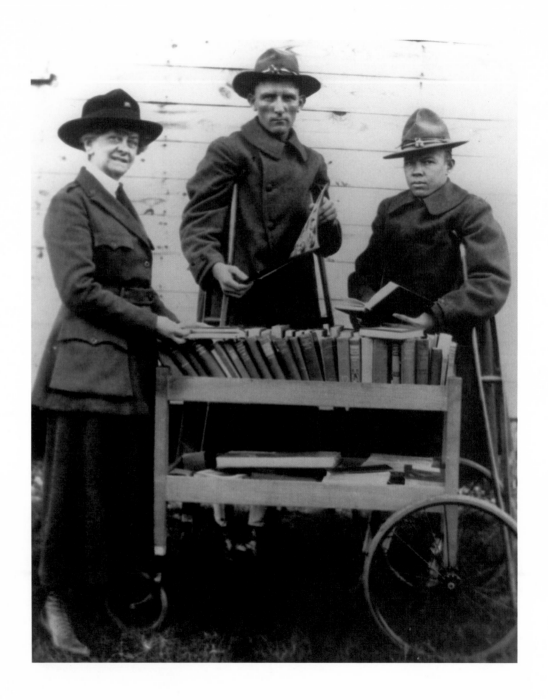

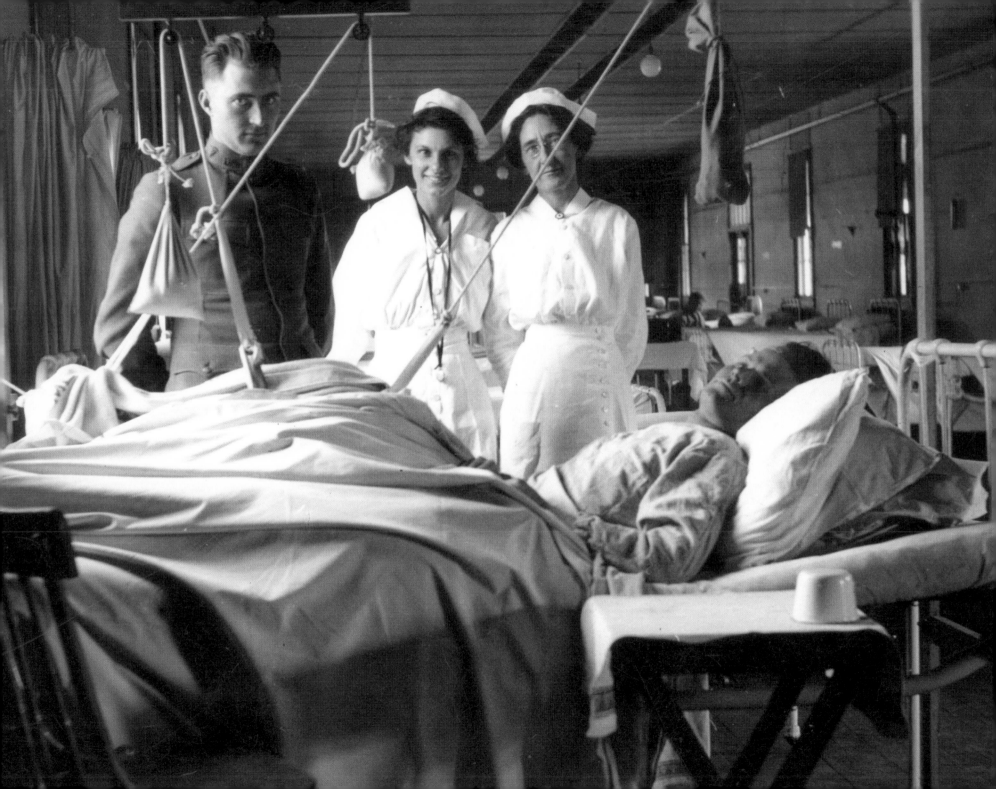

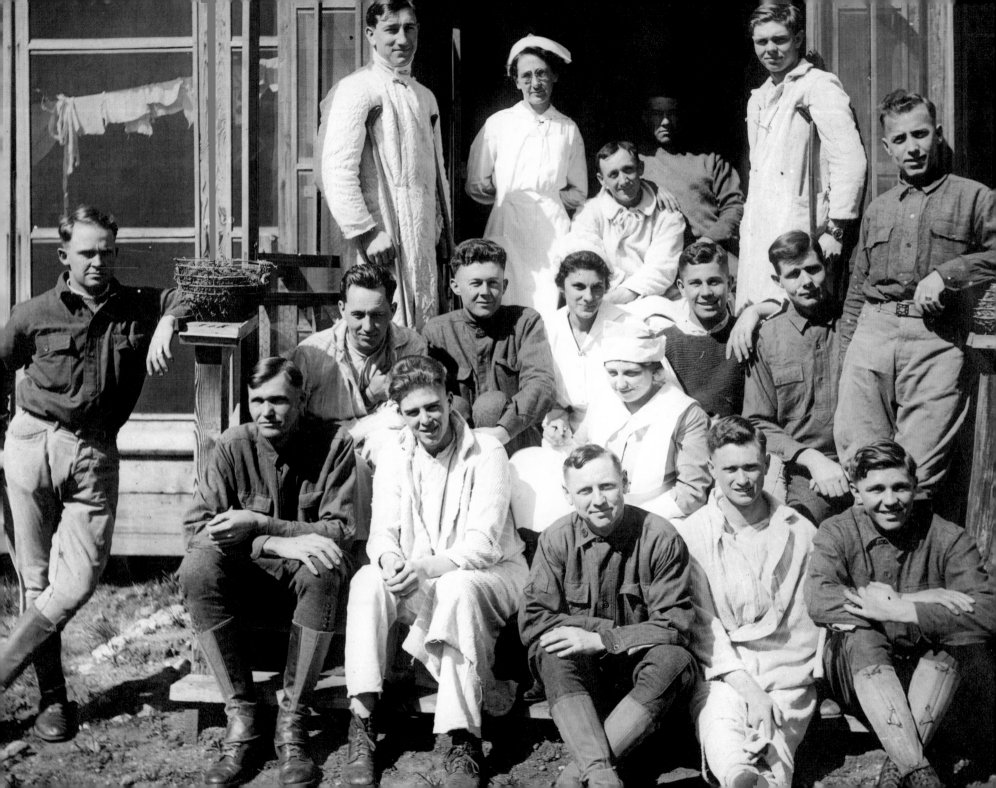

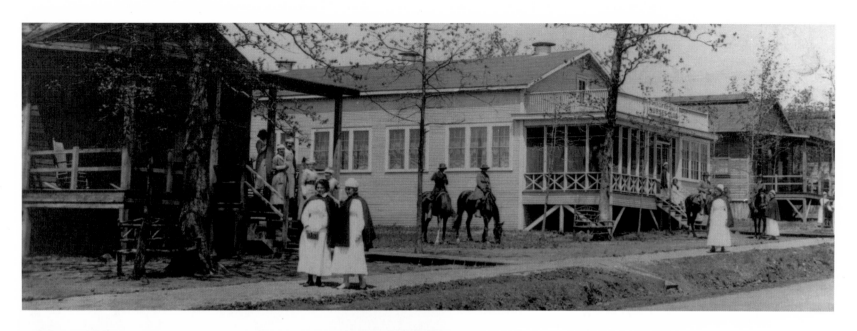

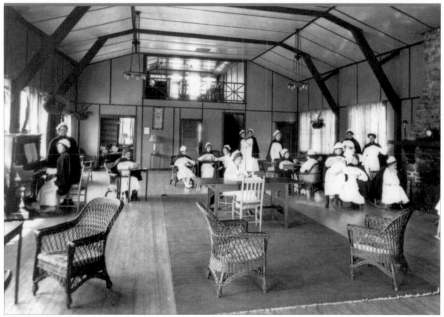

Camp Pike, located on a high, timbered, rolling plateau seven miles from Little Rock, Arkansas, received its first increment of drafted soldiers in September 1917. The men were quartered in frame barrack buildings. The incoming draft of July and August, 1918, filled the barracks to their capacity, thus necessitating the use of tents and sheds for the overflow.

(Opposite) *Patients on C-2 Ward, Camp Travis, Texas, February 20, 1918.*

(Right) *About 250 graduate nurses used these quarters and club at Camp Pike, Arkansas, during the war.*

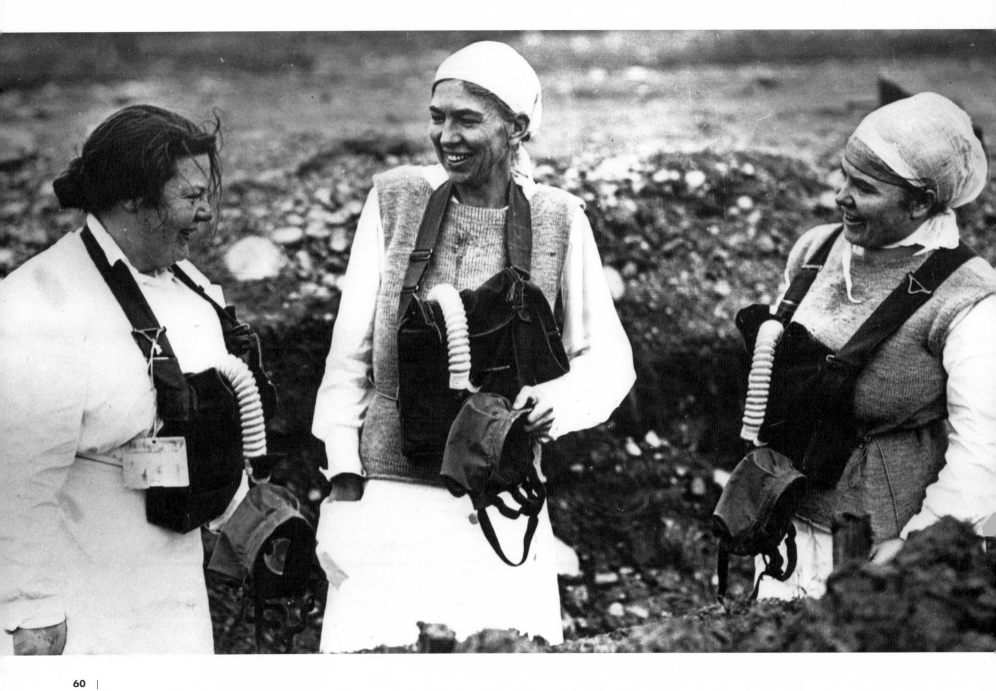

Training

ESTABLISHED JULY 18, 1917, Camp Kearny was located in southern California, 11 miles north of San Diego and 5 miles from the Pacific Ocean. It was one of 32 new camps created in May 1917, each designed to house 40,000 troops with 1,200 buildings and tents on 10,000 acres. Most of Camp Kearny's soldiers lived in tents, and more than 65,000 men passed through the camp on their way to World War I battlegrounds.

Some nurses received instruction in field operations before being sent to France. These photographs show nurses undergoing gas chamber training exercises at Camp Kearney, CA, March 30, 1918.

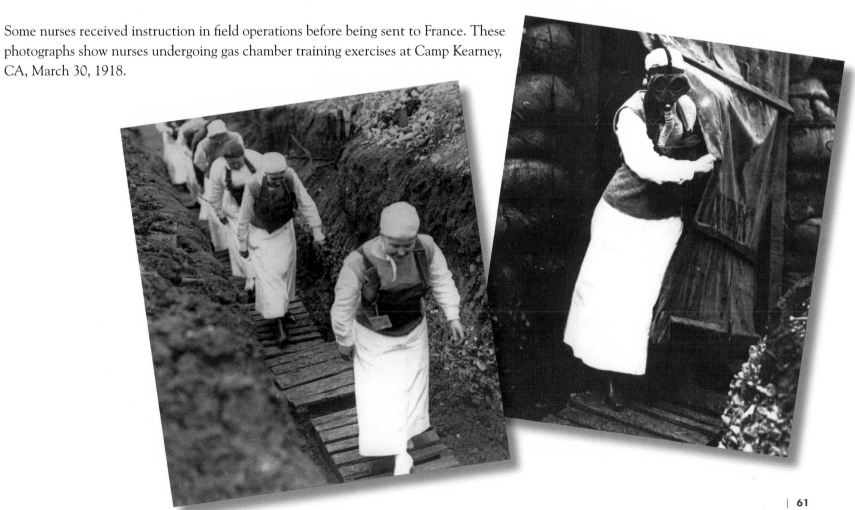

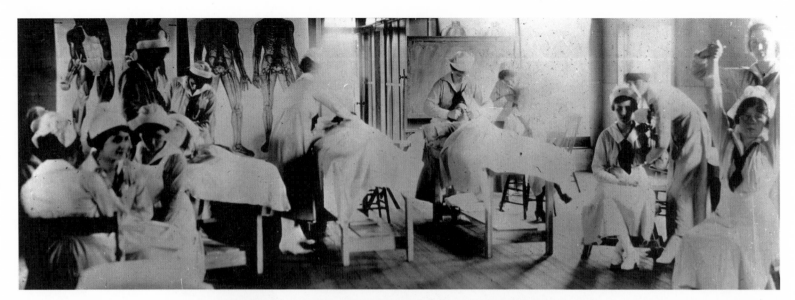

(Top) *Massage class and* (Bottom) *Riding class at Camp Sherman, Ohio, 1918.*

(Opposite) *Army and Red Cross nurses doing physical training in their white uniforms.*

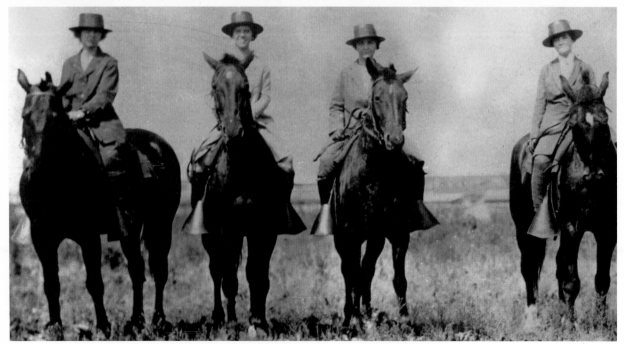

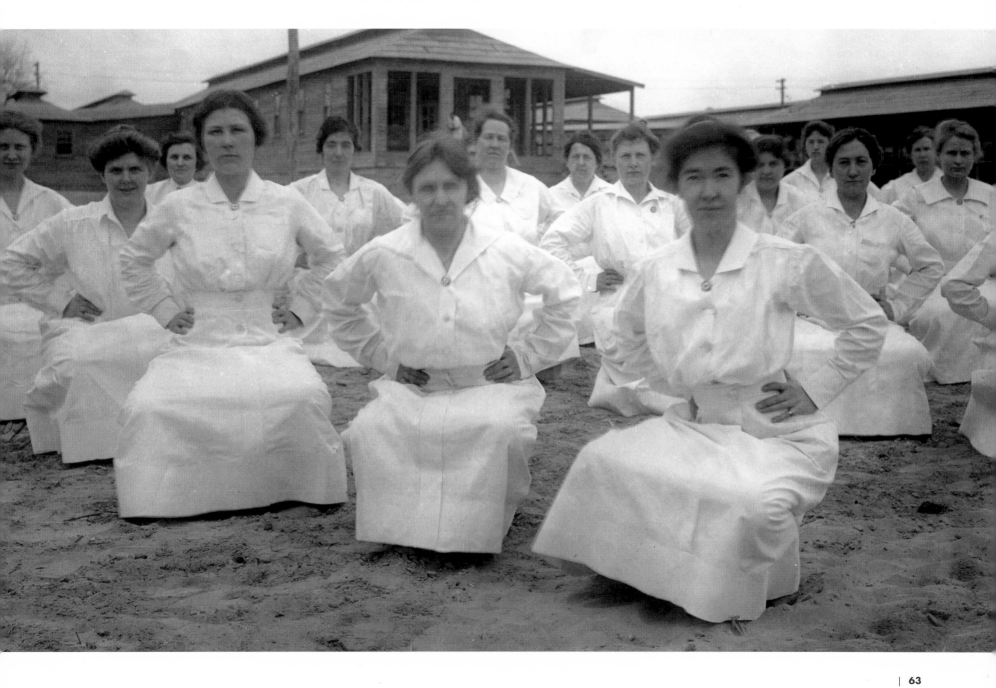

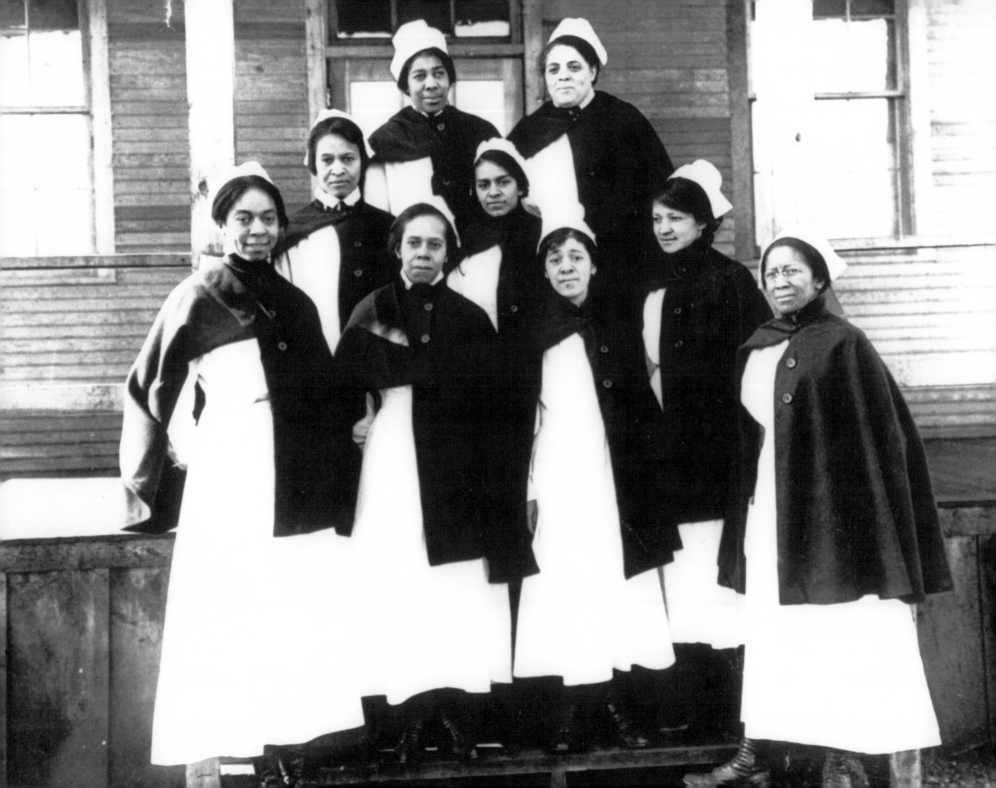

African American Nurses

BEFORE THE WAR, "NO COLORED NURSES had ever served in the Army Nurse Corps. Many of them, however, were anxious to join the corps if arrangements could be made, because of the relatively large number of colored troops in the Army…. In the fall of 1918 a few colored nurses were employed locally for emergencies at Camp Pike, Arkansas, and Camp Sevier, S.C." *(The Medical Dept in the World War, Vol. XIII, p. 292)*

African American nurses served in the ANC on a limited basis during the war after Jane Delano conferred with Superintendent Dora Thompson about accepting blacks into the organization. Thompson took the matter to the Surgeon General. He decided to enroll black nurses in the Red Cross reserve, but cautioned them not to expect a call to duty. The Army, which was segregated, cited the unavailability of the necessary quarters for black women as the rationale for their decision. In July 1918, plans to send groups of 20 black nurses to stations in the United States with large concentrations of black soldiers faltered due to delays in construction of separate quarters and mess facilities. Finally, the crisis of the influenza epidemic during the fall of 1918 precipitated the black nurses' entry into the Army Nurse Corps. However, it was not until after the armistice in December 1918 that these nurses actually came to serve. Nine nurses each cared for both black and white patients at Camp Sherman, Ohio, and Camp Grant, Illinois. *(Sarnecky, pp. 127–128)*

On the Battlefield

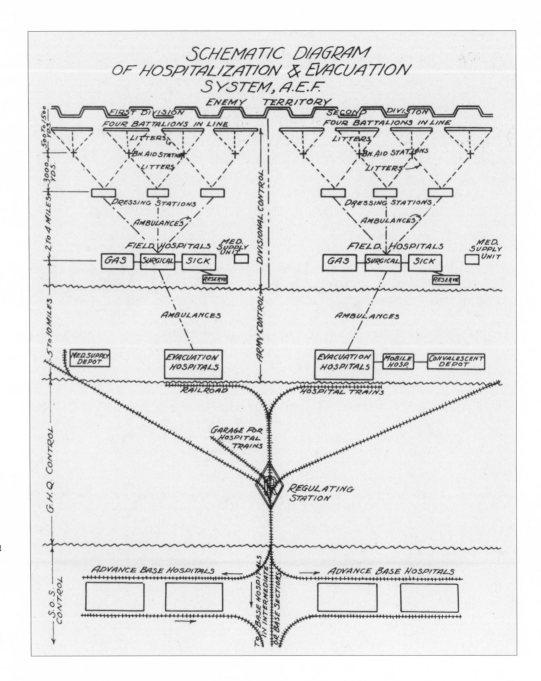

A schematic of doctrinally ideal evacuation from the battlefield. In practice, the American Expeditionary Forces (AEF) deviated from this model when the situation warranted.
(THE MEDICAL DEPT IN THE WORLD WAR, VOL. VIII, P. 262)

Buddy Aid

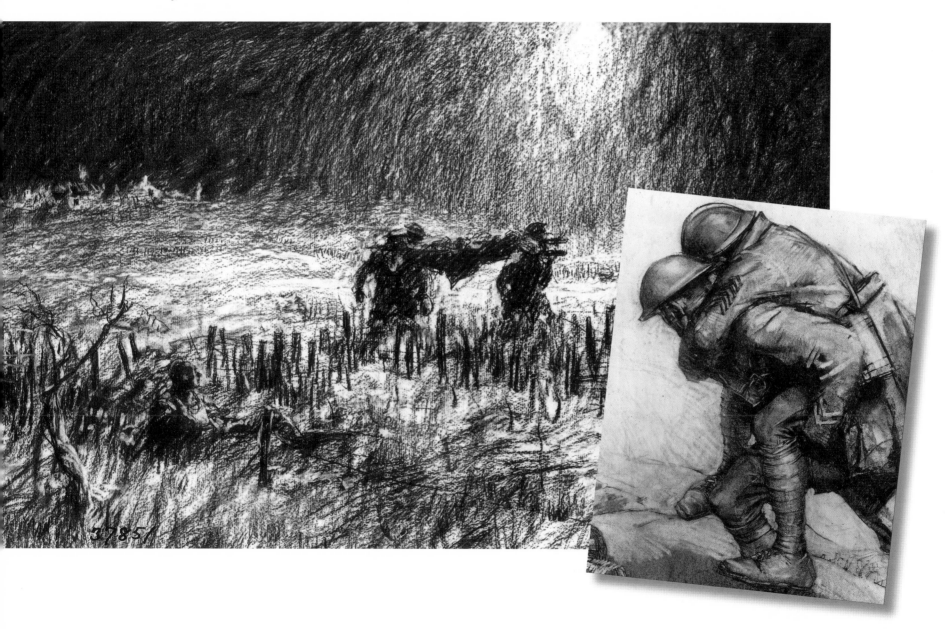

32851

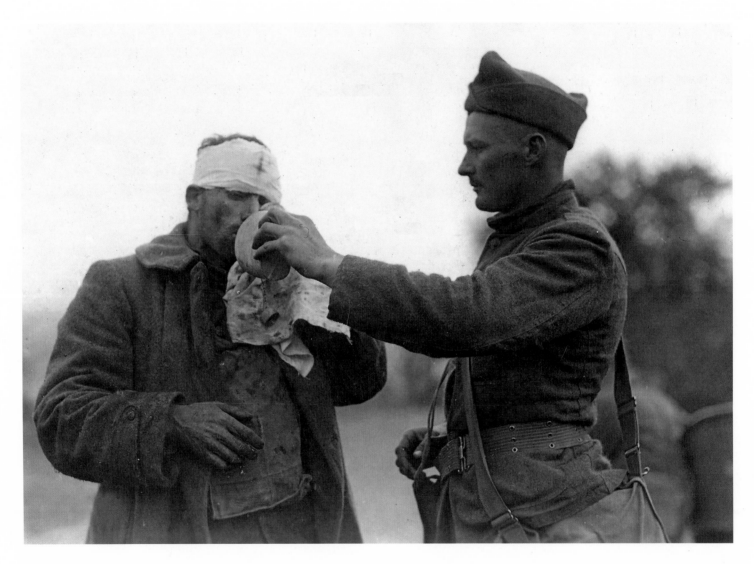

(Above) *Private John C. Jones, 61st Supply Company, giving a drink to a wounded comrade.*

Litter Bearers

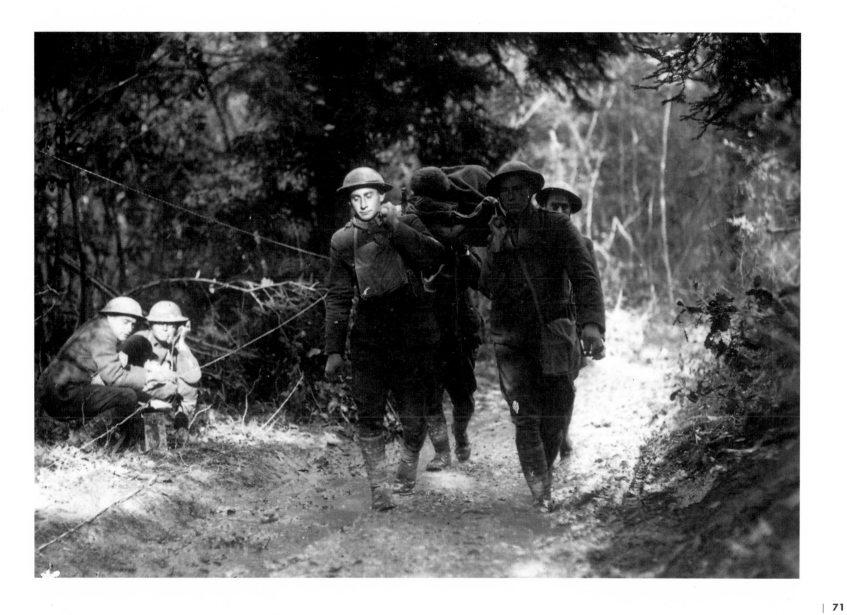

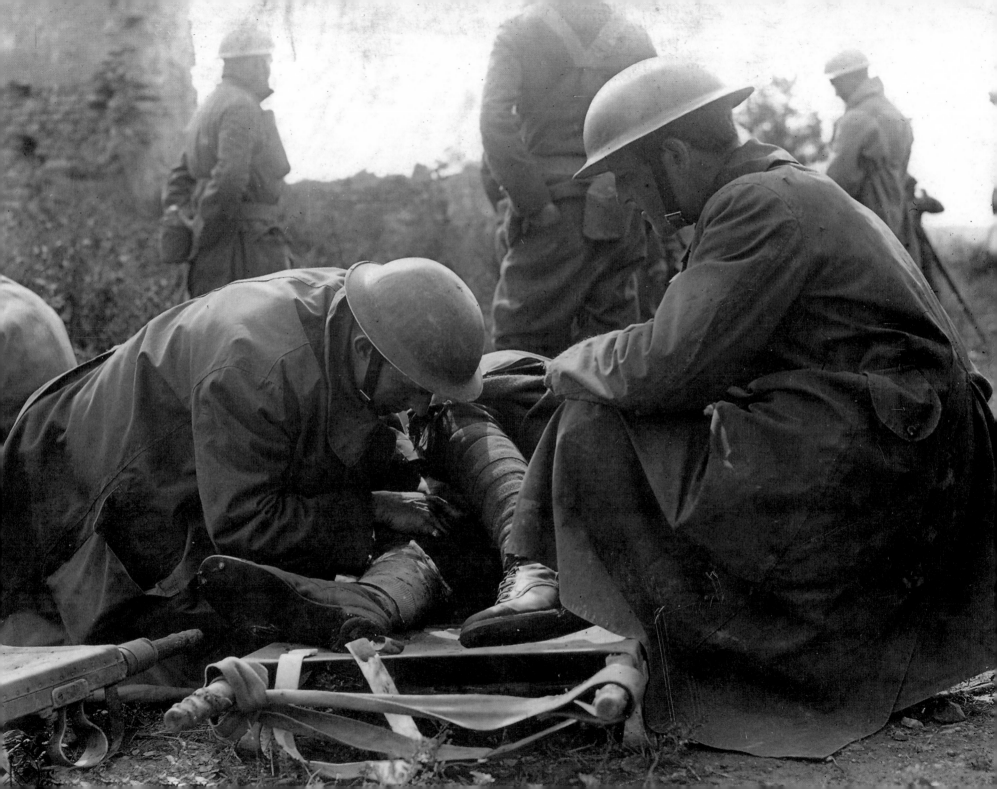

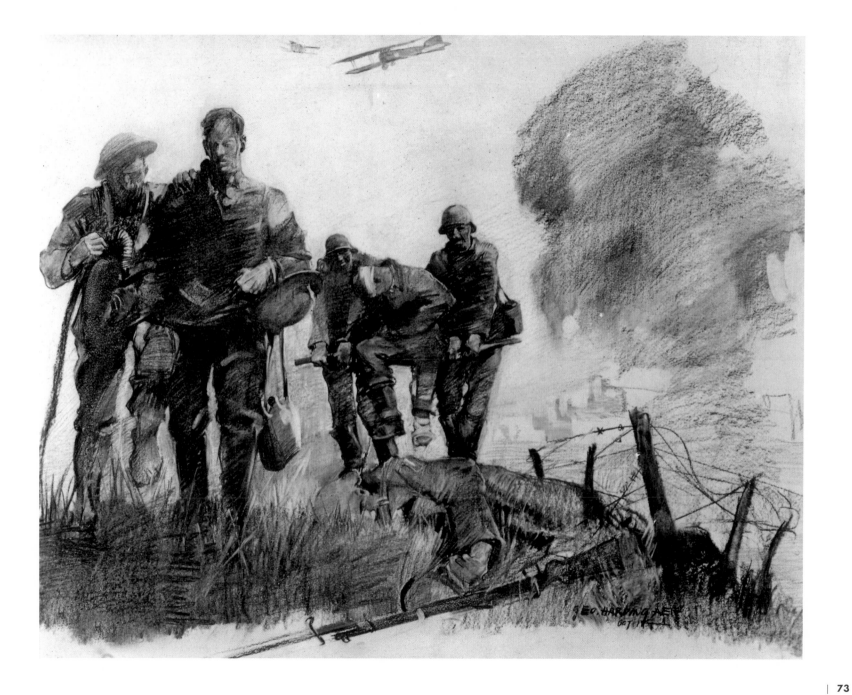

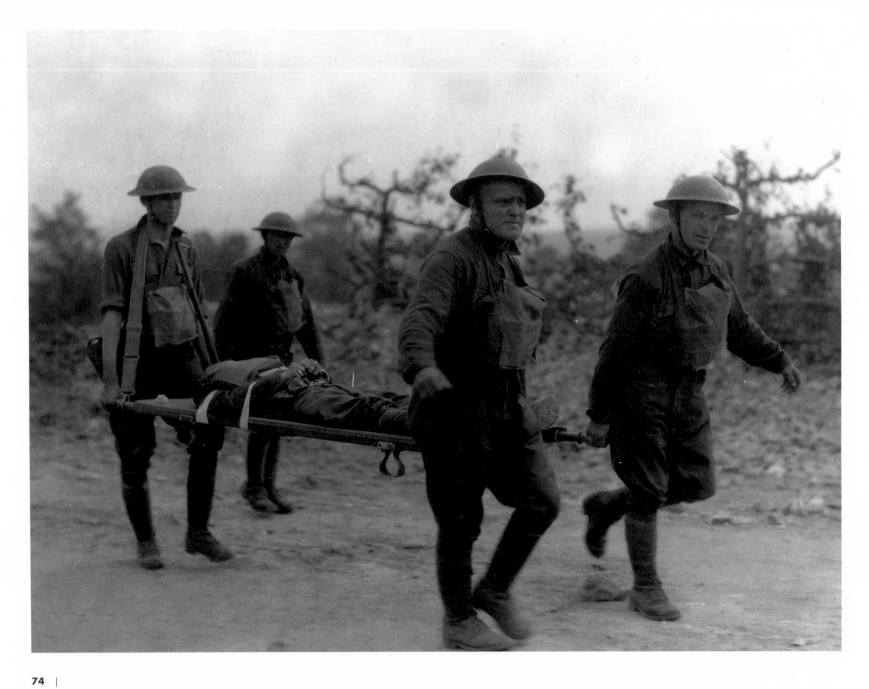

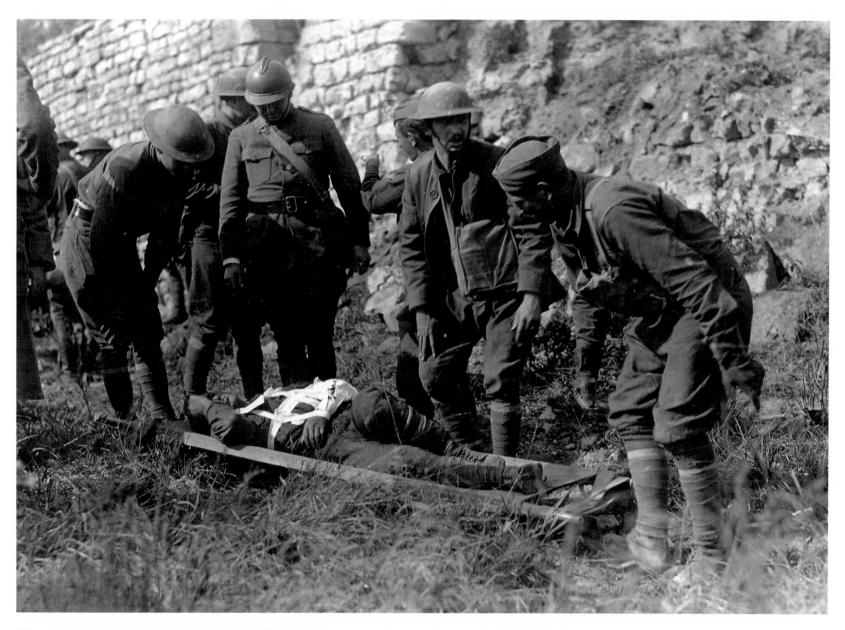

Wounded at first aid dressing station, Boureuilles, France.

Ambulances

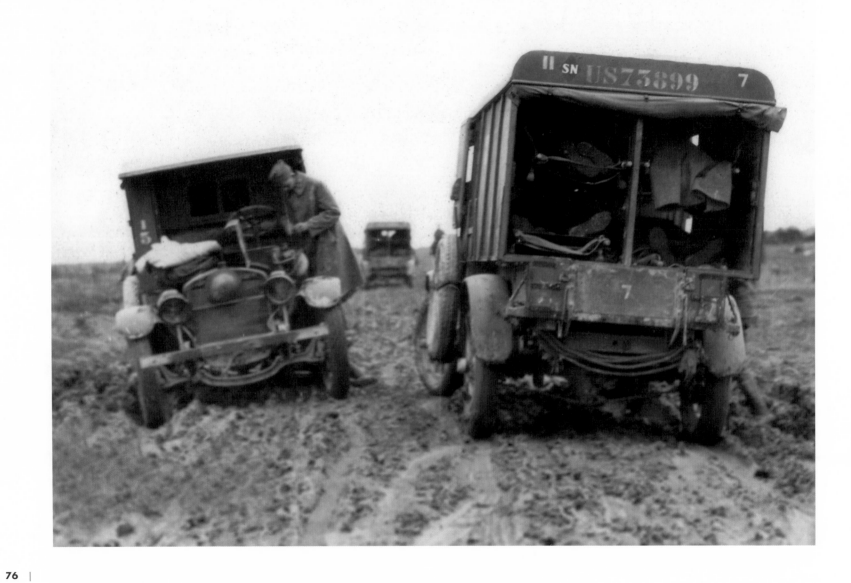

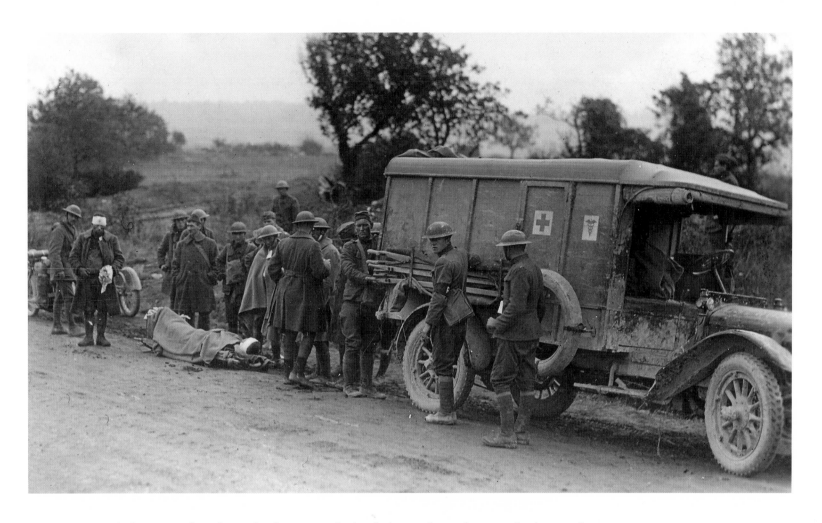

(Opposite) *Ambulances stuck in the mud. This is typical of ambulances driving between the front and evacuating stations. 5th Division, Meuse, France, October 13, 1918.*

(Above) *The 27th Ambulance Company of the 3rd Division receiving wounded on the outskirts of Nantillois, France. These men were gassed and wounded by shrapnel and machine gun fire. During the battle a constant stream of wounded were carried or helped to this station, where they were put in ambulances and rushed to hospitals. Many of these men are members of the 5th Division, which relieved the 80th Division, Nantillois, Meuse, France.*

(Left) *Rear view of ambulance with four wounded soldiers.*

(Opposite) *Wounded soldiers being transferred into ambulances.*

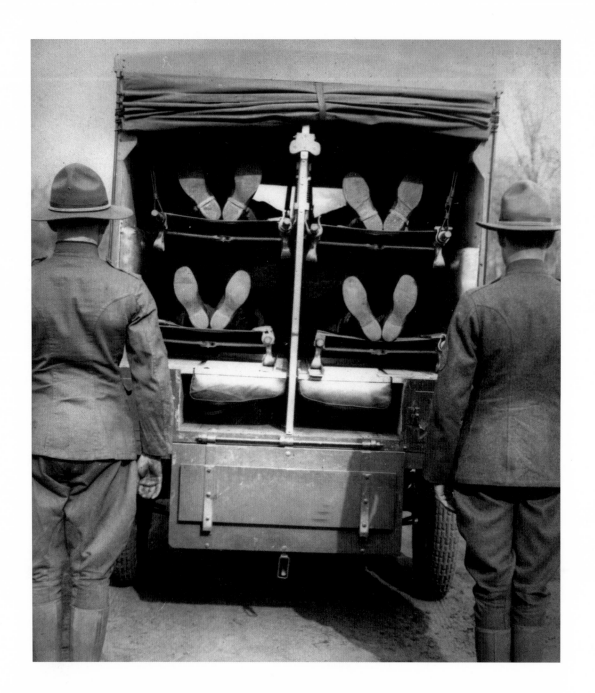

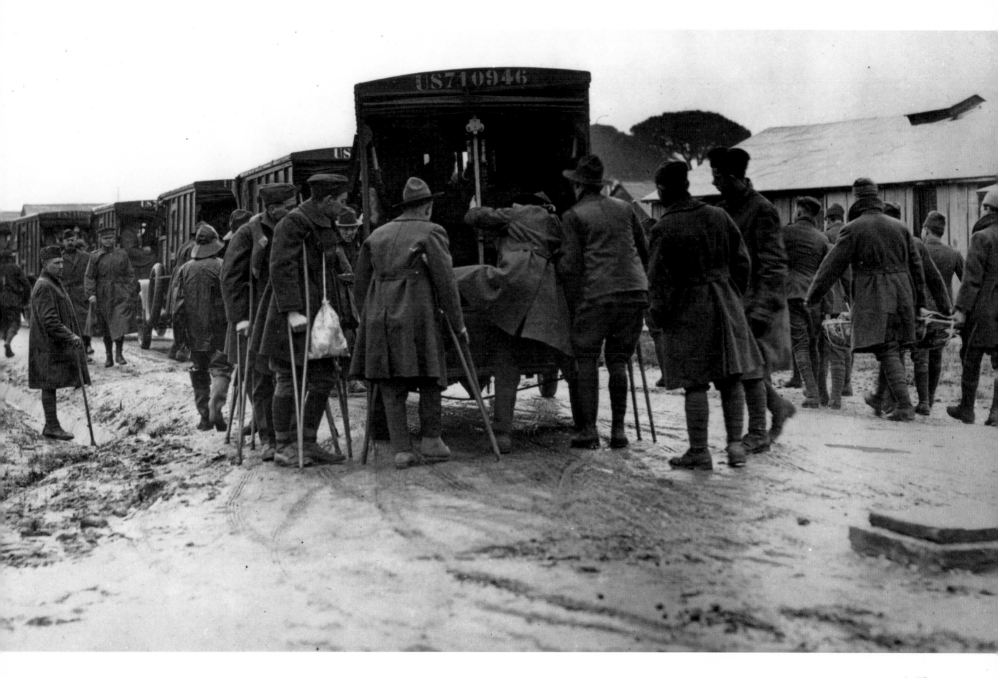

Field Hospitals

"NURSES WERE NOT INTENDED FOR ASSIGNMENT TO FIELD HOSPITALS, but there were occasions in which nurses found themselves on duty with such hospitals after having been assigned to duty on special surgical teams which were moved about as the need arose. Under such conditions formal reports of this service were never submitted, as there were no chief nurses on duty with these teams, but the nurses' individual records indicate that a number of nurses had varying lengths of service in connection with field hospitals." (*The Medical Dept in the World War, Vol. VIII, p. 335*)

❦❦

American Expeditionary Forces Medical Specialty Teams—One method whereby Army nurses moved from the rear areas to the front lines was as members of special teams. These five- or six-person teams were a new doctrinal concept that enabled the AEF to quickly move highly specialized health care providers to specific areas of the battlefield where they were most needed. Typical teams included shock, surgical, gas, and orthopedic teams.

The primary function of shock teams was the resuscitation of wounded soldiers who were unstable due to blood loss, usually as a result of a femur fracture or multiple trauma, and therefore too ill to survive immediate surgery. Treatments typically consisted of intravenous administration of whole blood and fluids.

Many nurses also served as members of surgical teams. These teams were specially trained to care for immediate surgical, neurosurgical, orthopedic, maxillofacial and chest cases. In addition to traditional roles, nurses served as anesthetists on the teams. By operating on wounded soldiers right at the front instead of forcing them to endure a lengthy evacuation process, these teams proved invaluable for decreasing morbidity and mortality.

Gas teams provided care to patients who survived gas attacks. Care was largely supportive and consisted of rest, morphine, oxygen, and stimulants. Removal of exudate from the lungs was accomplished by inducing vomiting and later by the use of benzoin steam tents.

These roles were revolutionary, exposing women to danger by bringing them closer to the front then ever before. Women readily volunteered to serve with these teams rather than remain back in the rear where it was safe. In the words of Julia Stimson, being chosen to move forward was "the goal and prize for which every nurse . . . longed."

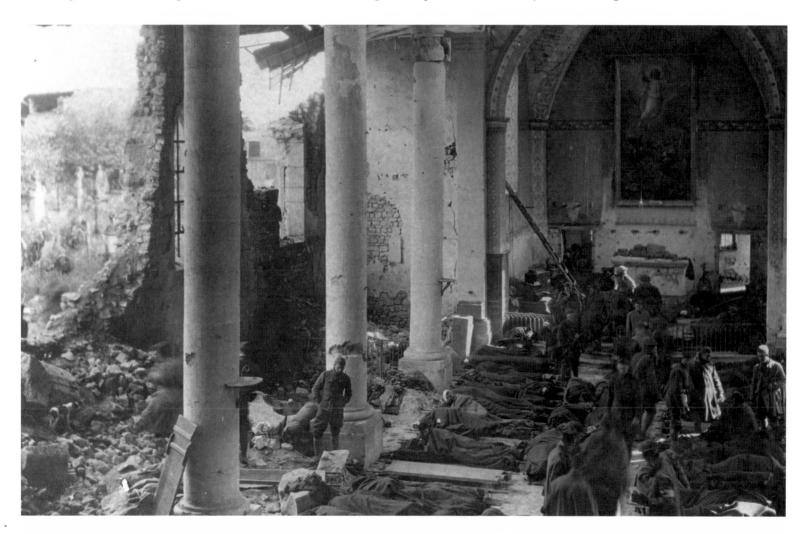

Soldiers wounded in action receiving medical treatment in an old, war-battered church, by personnel of the 110th Sanitary Train, Field Hospital No. 137, 35th Division, Neuilly, Meuse, France. September 29, 1918.

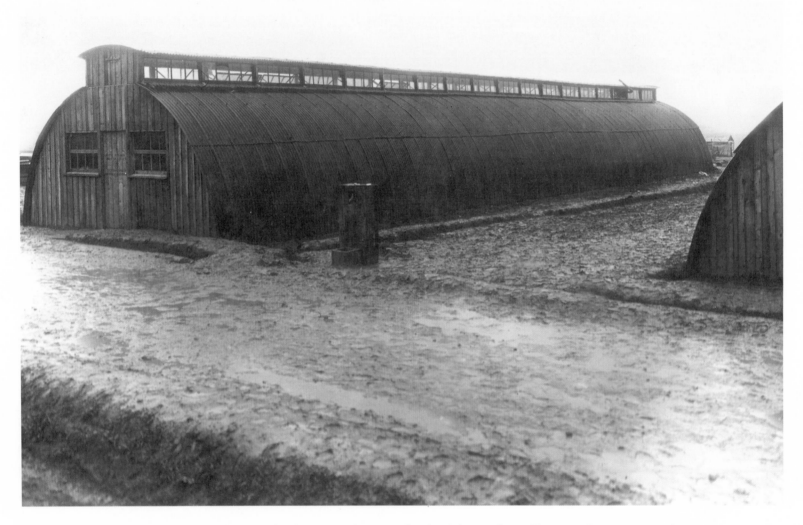

One of the buildings made of corrugated iron used as bunk house, for Field Hospitals Nos. 138 and 139, near Vertuzey, Meuse, France. December 1918.

Mobile Hospitals

MOBILE SURGICAL HOSPITALS, usually established in tents, were organizations destined for activity near the front lines. These hospitals were forced to move on very short notice, so their personnel had to be skilled in rapidly erecting and taking down tents. They augmented other hospitals, especially evacuation hospitals, during major operations involving many casualties.

Mobile surgical hospitals had complete equipment for operations, their own laundries, sterilizing trucks, and electric-lighting plants. Many of them had portable equipment on trucks that could be incorporated into a tent system and function as a room. For instance, X-ray and sterilizing trucks could be attached to the operating room. All the equipment could be taken down, packed into trucks, transported a considerable distance, and set up again on the same day.

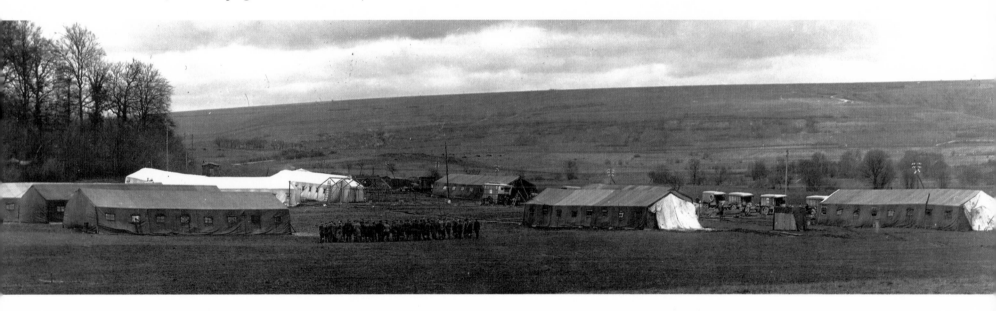

Panoramic view of Mobile Hospital No. 39 near Chalons-sur-Marne in the St. Mihiel sector, Meuse, France. This hospital handled the left sector of St. Mihiel drive, including the II and IV Corps of the Second Army. December 1918.

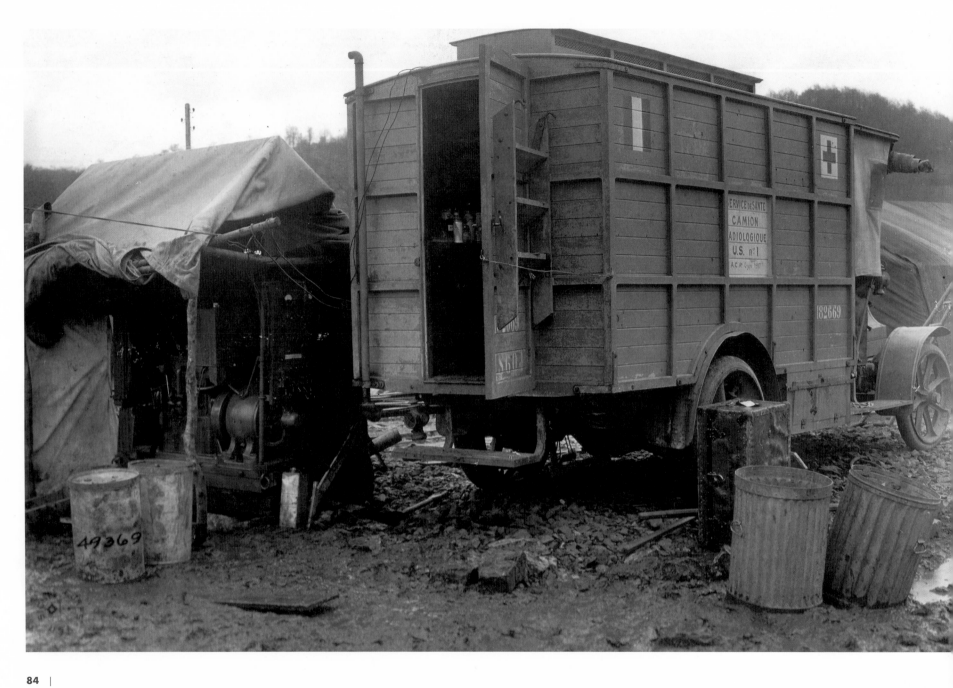

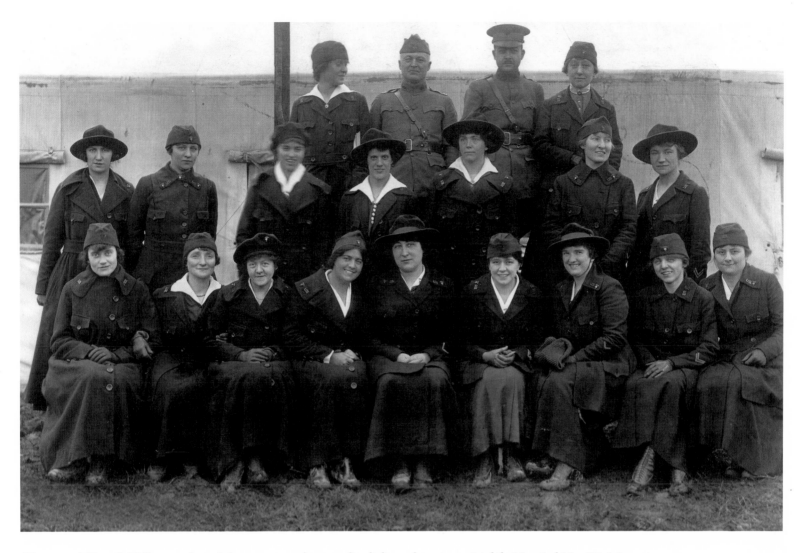

(Opposite) *French X-Ray truck and the generator that supplies light to the tents at Mobile Hospital No. 39, Meuse, France. December 1918.*

(Above) *Nurse staff of Mobile Hospital No. 39. Effie M. White (head nurse); Captain Grant Augustine and Lieutenant R.S. Elliston, at top of group, Meuse, France. December 19, 1918.*

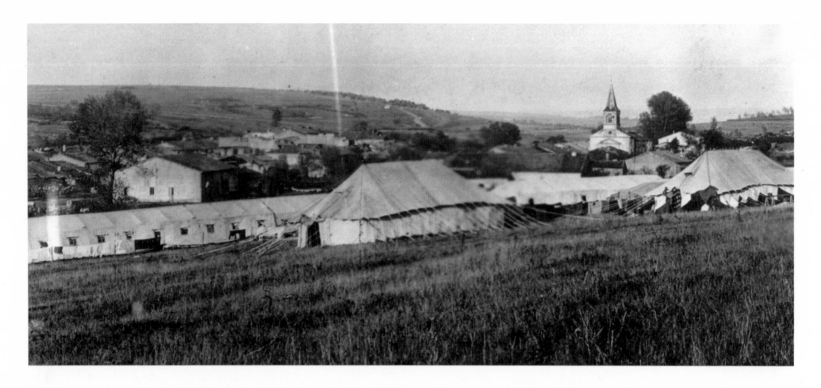

Mobile hospital staff usually included 20 nurses, or 19 nurses and the chief nurse. Conditions were necessarily primitive. A special tent was used for the nurses' quarters, usually containing little more than beds and locker trunks, which held all the nurses' necessities inside and their wash basins and pitchers on top. The mess tent usually contained trestles with boards for tables and benches for chairs. If oilcloth was available it was used for table covering, and dishes consisted of easily transportable enamel plates and bowls. Because screens and mosquito netting could not be installed in these rapidly moving units, flies caused much annoyance. In some mobile hospitals recreation tents for the nurses' use were provided by the American Red Cross.

(Above) *View of 1st Mobile Hospital, III Army Corps, Fromerville, Meuse, France, October 22, 1918. The commanding officer of Mobile Hospital No. 1 also served as Director of Surgery for Evacuation Hospital No. 7.*

(Opposite) *Group of nurses at Mobile Hospital No. 2, Auteuil, Paris, July 1, 1918.*

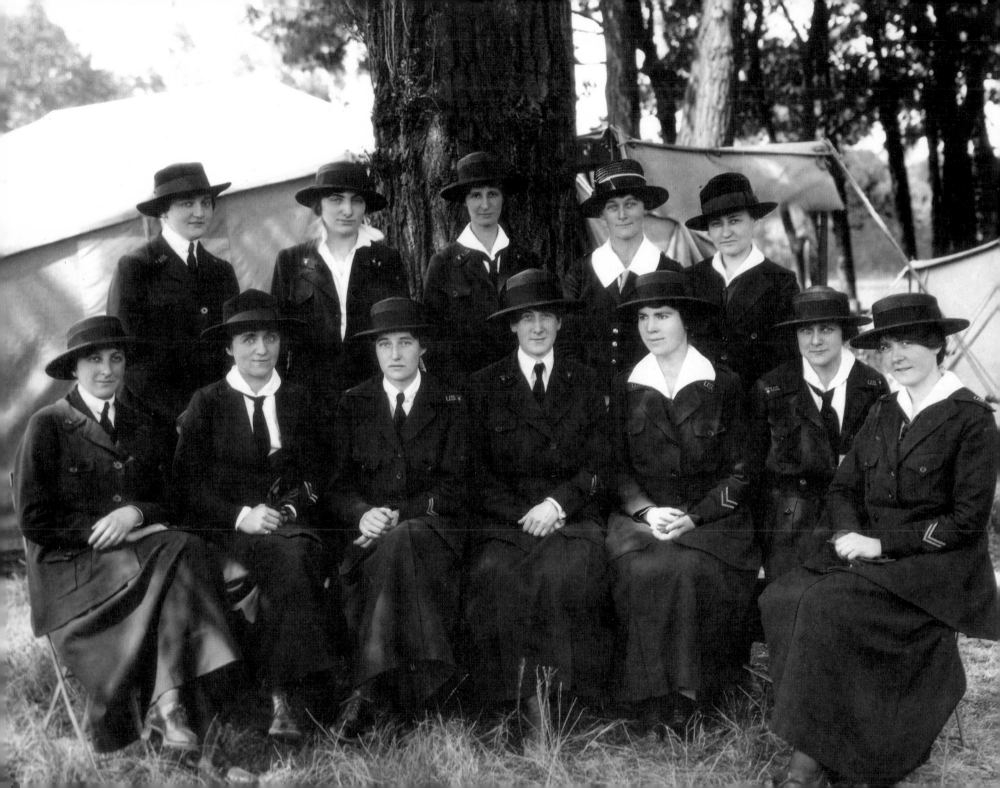

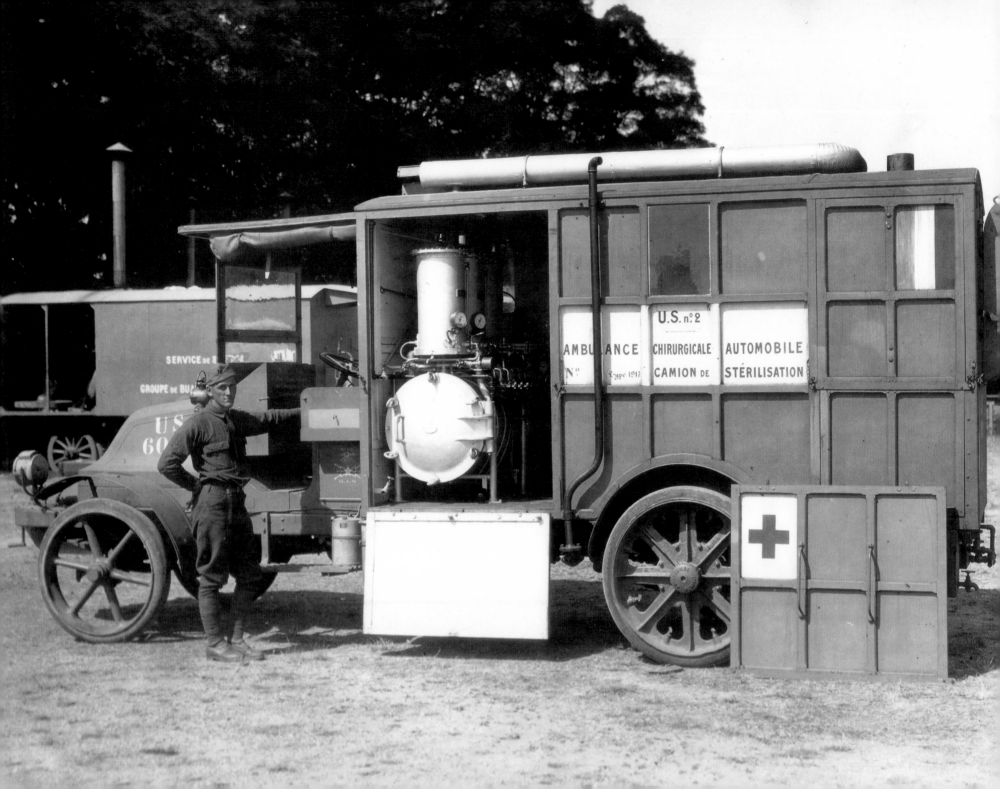

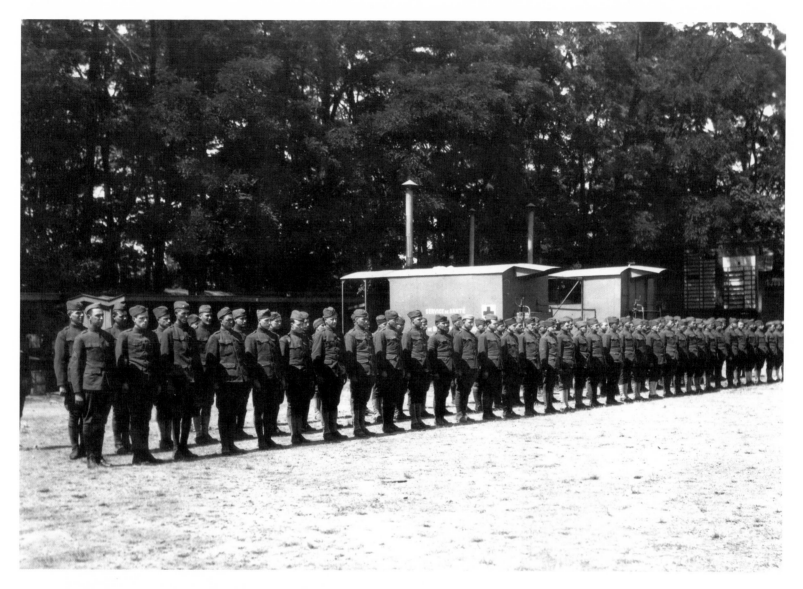

(Opposite) *Sterilizer truck at Auteuil, Paris, Mobile Hospital No. 2.*

(Above) *Group of enlisted men at Mobile Hospital No. 2.*

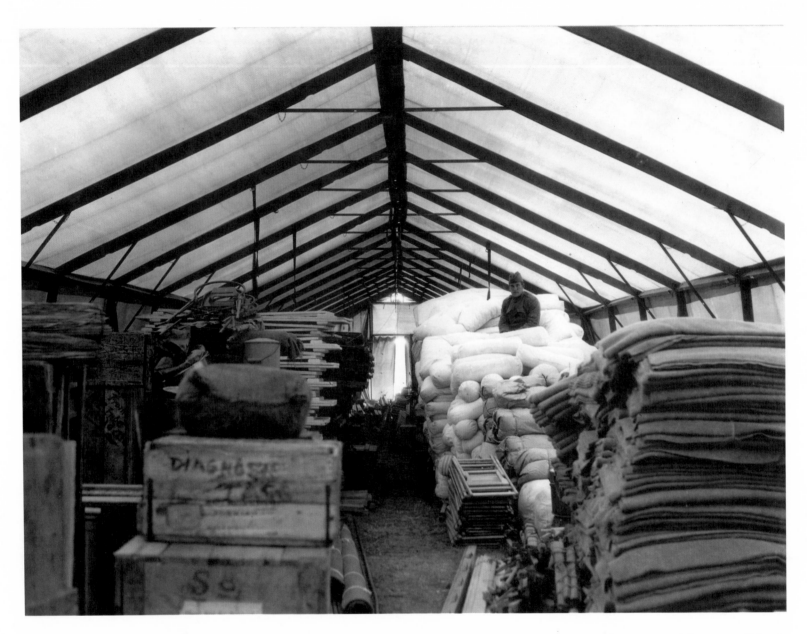

Interior of the supply tent at Mobile Hospital No. 2.

Evacuating the Wounded

"OWING TO THE EXTREME CONGESTION and violent shelling of all roads and to terrific machine-gun fire in the front lines, it was oftentimes impossible to remove the wounded until dark.

"Roads were constantly jammed with divisions taking their places in the line, and the divisions which were being relieved moving back. Some effort was made to reserve certain roads for evacuation of the wounded, but it was apparently impossible. In spite of these conditions, however, the average length of time in transporting a wounded man from the place of receiving his wound to the field hospital consumed a period between 3 to 8 hours. The evacuation hospitals . . . were so far to the rear that no average time could be calculated for the transportation of the wounded to those points. At the beginning of the Argonne drive evacuation hospitals were from 30 to 60 kilometers from the field hospitals." *(Surgeon General Report, 1919, Vol. II)*

"I have never in all my life seen such tenderness as these men show to each other. If you could see, as we so often see, men with horrible leg injuries reaching way over to feed the man in the bed next to them, who may have arm injuries and be helpless. And always the up-patients are so good to the bed-ridden ones. Our hospital simply could not run without the help of the patients themselves. They fetch and carry and bathe and scrub and hold legs and arms for dressings, and joke and jolly each other along till it would break your heart, for they themselves are sick men." *(October 14, 1917, Stimson, Finding Themselves, p. 139)*

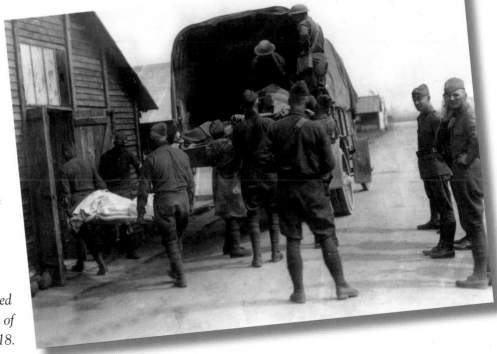

Unloading a truck at Field Hospital No. 326, filled with gassed men of the 82nd and 89th Divisions, north of Royaumeix, France. October 15, 1918.

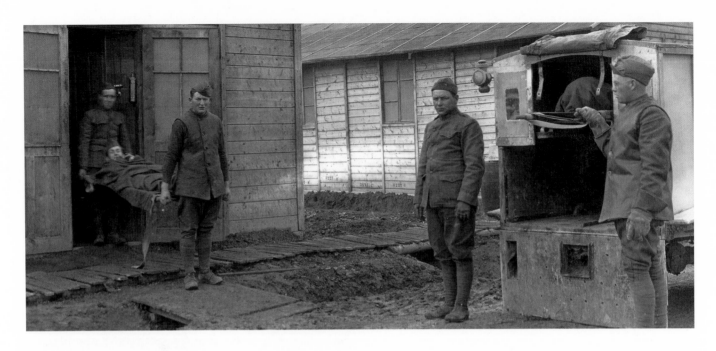

"Saturday—we received our first real convoy, about 300 all 42nd Div . . . I received 68 on my floor, mostly mustard gas burns, terrific suffering. The convoy arrived about 6:00 PM. I worked until 10:30 trying to get them settled." *(March 23, 1918, Maude Frances Essig)*

"Sunday—what a change from last week. 82 patients on my floor, about 20 doctors assigned to my floor. All want something, every place. Stat. We do not have supplies nor equipment to meet their demands, this type of burn is terrible and nothing seems to give relief. Eye and genitalia burns are the most painful, terrible situation. The patients are good scouts, and most appreciative. So happy to be in the hands of USA." *(March 24, 1918, Maude Frances Essig)*

(Above) *Gassed patients of the 82nd and 89th Divisions being loaded into U.S. ambulances at Field Hospital No. 326, north of Royaumeix, France.*

(Opposite) *General scene of evacuation, Base Hospitals No. 88 and No. 53. Langres, Haute Marne, France.*

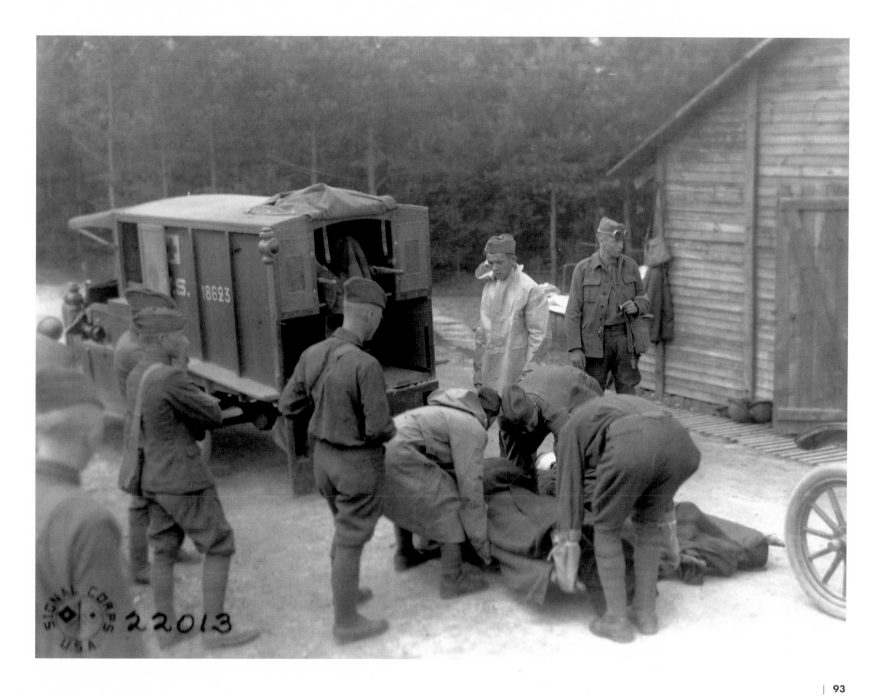

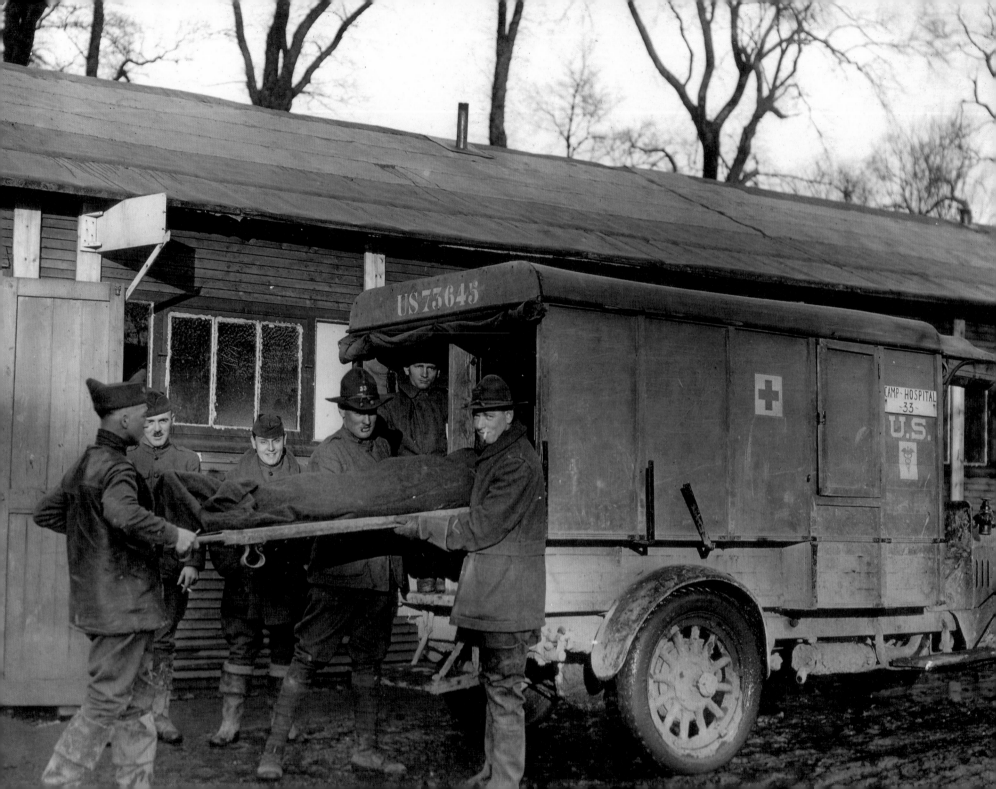

"Experience demonstrated that five different groups of bearers were necessary: (1) Four men to unload ambulances and carry patients to the bathing tables; (2) four men to carry patients to the X-ray room; (3) a supervisor and four men to handle patients in the X-ray room; (4) a supervisor and six men to remove patients from operating tables and carry them to wards; (5) eight men for evacuating patients. One supervisor and one man were required to remove soiled litters and blankets from the admission room. For a 500-bed hospital, running 6 double teams continuously, two shifts of 28 men each were required. The nature of the work was such that 8-hour periods proved better than those of 12 hours." *(The Medical Dept in the World War, Vol. VIII, p. 198)*

✂✂

"The transport and hospitalization of the sick and wounded of the American Expeditionary Forces, after [they] had been evacuated from the zone of the armies, presented difficulties which differed in many respects from those which had confronted the French army during three and a half years of warfare, and also from those of the British, whose system of evacuation was similar to that of the French though modified by geographical conditions. The French and British systems involved no long lines of communications to home ports. The short route to England made it possible for British wounded to reach home bases rapidly.

The American Army, however, was compelled to hospitalize in France, and to some extent in England, almost all its sick and wounded, since it was impracticable to send home any except a relatively small number, who were permanently (from a military viewpoint) disabled. To meet the needs imposed by this situation and to economize on personnel and materiel, the American Expeditionary Forces had recourse to the use of large hospitals and hospital groups into which patients could be received by the trainload. These organizations necessarily were situated on supply lines of the American Expeditionary Forces." *(The Medical Dept in the World War, Vol. VIII, p. 261)*

(Opposite) *Unloading patients from ambulances, Camp Hospital No. 33, Brest, Finistere, France.*

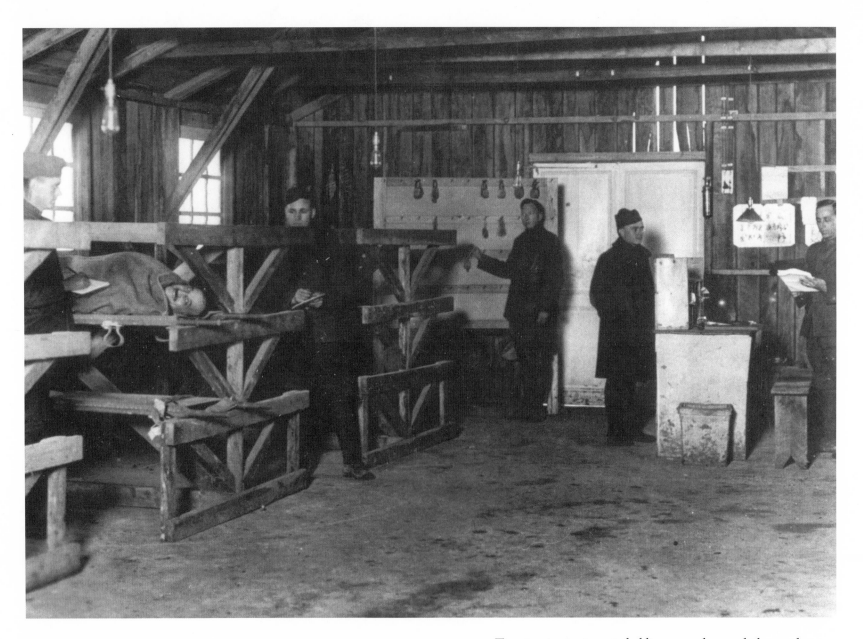

Transporting patients in holding area, date and place unknown.

Evacuation Hospitals

AEF EVACUATION HOSPITALS had between 1,000 and 1,500 beds. Under ideal conditions the hospitals were located at a rail head within from eight to ten miles of the front, so that the wounded could arrive rapidly by ambulance and either be operated on immediately or sent by train to hospitals to the rear. From the nursing point of view, however, little functional difference existed between evacuation and base hospitals, except that the turnover of their patients was generally more rapid. *(The Medical Dept in the World War, Volume VIII, p. 334)*

"These hospitals are the backbone of all combat hospitalization." *(Surgeon General Report, 1919, Vol. II, p. 1465)*

"Tell Papa that living in these Evacuation Hospitals at the front has camping in the Maine wood skun a hundred way [*sic*]. It is so much worse. In Maine woods you can cut enough wood to keep warm where over here if you cut down any trees the French have a fit about it, and the coal they have isn't any good. It is just like dust." *(November 30, 1918, Elizabeth Lewis, Vichy, France)*

❧❧

"I don't know hardly what to write about up here as there isn't [*sic*] any French people or any stories or in fact we are the only women around here. I will be glad when I get back to civilization so I can have some where to go, all there is here is a shell torn village which has been desserted [*sic*] for a long time. All there is here is soldiers. It seems so queer to be in a place where no one lives around. This trip has been a great experience to me, and also a great sight seeing trip, I am glad I have had it but one of these is enough for me. If I ever get back to the base they will never get me on another operating team. I will tell them to send some one out that hasn't had a trip. They are living at the base [Base Hospital No. 15] in a swell hotel and having their pay and mail regular, and a fine city to live in. Our base is really in best place I have been in France. Here we are out on these teams never getting any mail or never have been payed, [*sic*] and are pounced around from place to place. Never knowing from one meal to the next where we will be." *(Elizabeth Lewis, Army Nurse Corps, attached to American Red Cross Hospital No.110 on night operating shift.)*

"I have had the privilege of being with the nearest Evacuation hospital to the lines. This is the nearest nurses have ever been to the front. I didn't want to tell you while the war was on for I knew you would worry. I will tell you now though. We had to have our gas masks with us all the time, and there [were] a few nights I wore my helmet back and forth to midnight lunch. When you see the shells whizzing all around you that is as near the front as I want to get. I must admit I was crazy to get near the front but I have had my desire satisfied here. Fortunately no one was injured at the hospital, but in the village a few yards from us two men were injured one day and in the city the Germans were always throwing over gas as shells, and I tell you this has been quite an exsighting [*sic*] place here." *(November 13, 1918, Elizabeth Lewis)*

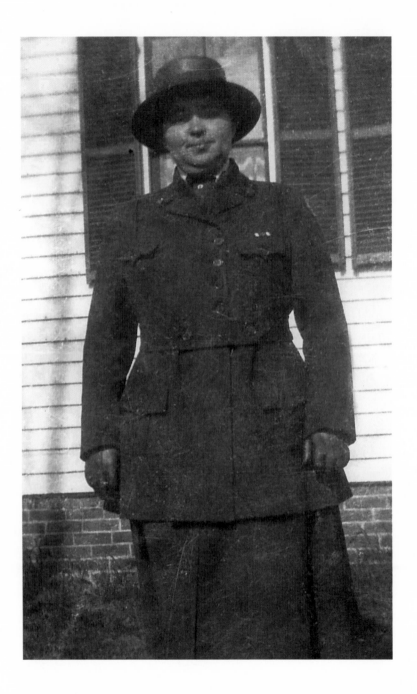

(Left) *Army nurse Elizabeth Lewis, attached to Evacuation Hospital No. 15.* (Photograph courtesy of the Army Heritage Center Foundation)

(Opposite) *Destruction of Ward No. 2, Bussy-le-Chateau, Marne, by six-inch shell, killing two men. American nurses survived unscathed. July 17, 1918.*

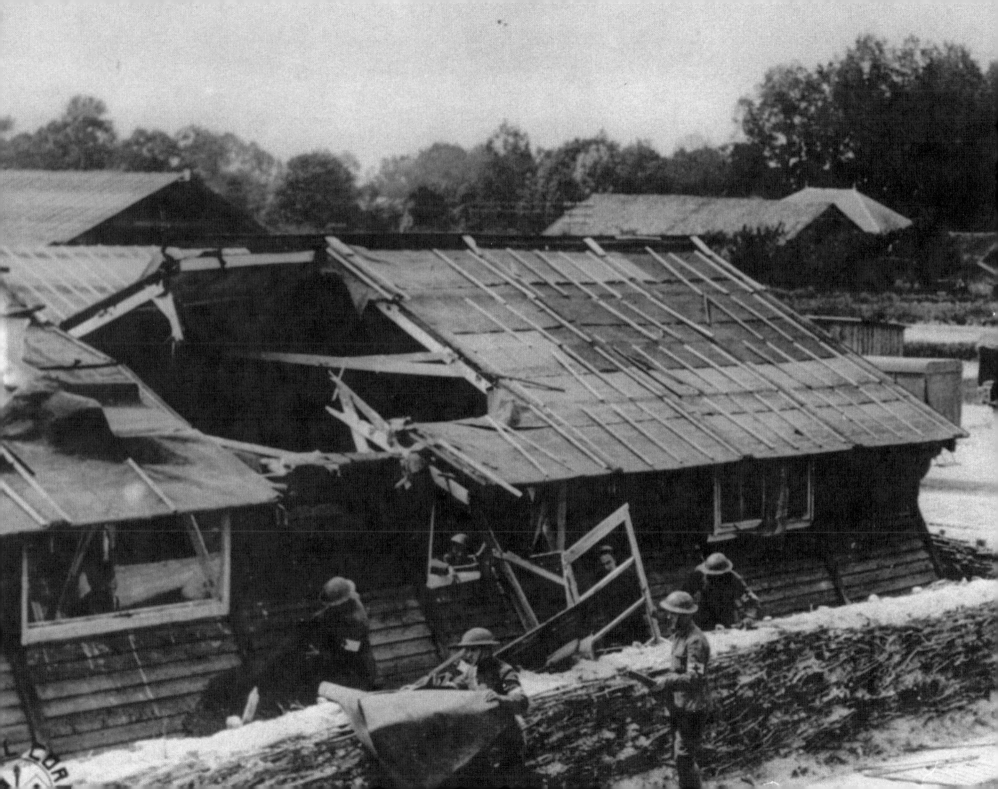

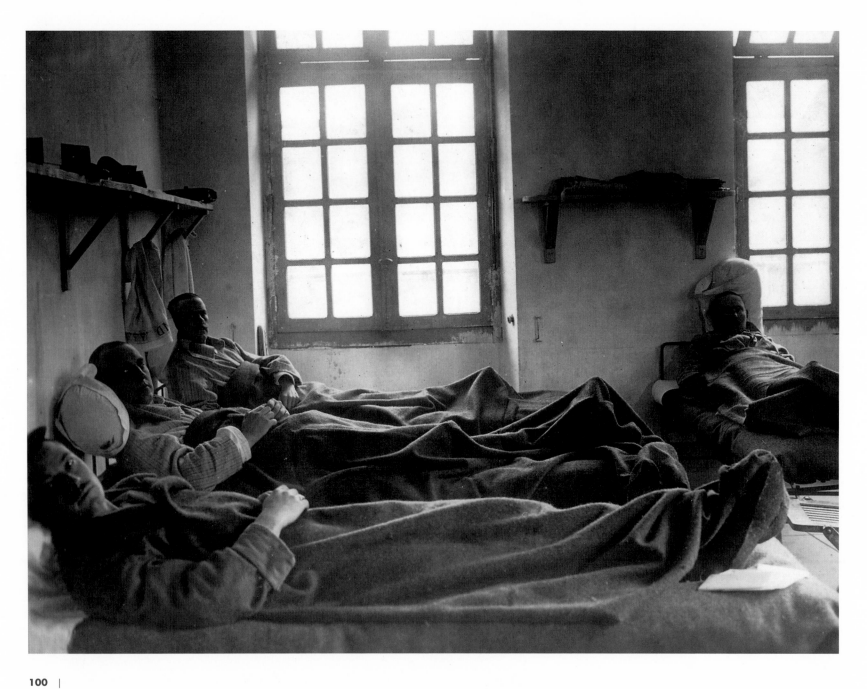

"My children at the front are having such wonderful times. They are working terribly hard, sleeping with helmets over their faces and enamel basins on their stomachs, washing in the water they had in their hot-water bags because water is so scarce, operating fourteen hours at a stretch, drinking quantities of tea because there is no coffee and nothing else to drink, wearing men's ordnance socks under their stockings, trying to keep their feet warm in the frosty operating rooms at night, and both seeing and doing such surgical work as they never in their wildest days dreamed of, but all the time unafraid and unconcerned with the whistling, banging shells exploding around them. Oh, they are fine! One need never tell me that women can't do as much, stand as much, and be as brave as men." *(October 9, 1917, Stimson, Finding Themselves, p. 134)*

❧❧

"We are very busy, all beds are filled and every staff member is working the limit. The stretcher bearers are working very hard, they have to carry the patients up the 8 flights of stairs, then down 7 flights to operating rooms and back up the 7 flights to bed. I surely pity them. Also we need more orderlies, the sickest patients are kept on the lower floors but we have plenty who are very sick and we have more to do then [sic] we can get done, our census today is 130 on my floor, I shudder where I have time to think of what they have been through, the patients are all cheerful and so glad to have such a 'swell place,' many are lying on straw ticks on the floor, much better than lying out on the battlefield waiting for some one to rescue them, they say. Last night 14 of my patients went to surgery, three surgical teams worked all night, my patients were all back from surgery by 11 PM and it meant a busy night for me and my one orderly, all patients had eaten red beans for supper, and had ether anesthesia on full stomach, so we had some really sick boys until the red beans were eliminated." *(July 24, 1918, Maude Frances Essig)*

(Opposite) *Officers' convalescent ward, American Evacuation Hospital, No. 2, Baccarat, France. May 10, 1918.*

"Our census increases day by day. We receive and evacuate every other day, more arrive than are sent away, my floor is fairly quiet after mid-night. Most of the patients sleep through Dakin irrigations, yet when they are awake they fuss considerably about treatments. Last Thursday we received a large convoy at an early morning hour and we stayed on duty until after our evening meal. That evening 16 of our patients went to surgery, no operating done after 11 PM. These are busy nights and busier days . . . our patients are coming directly from The Front and they say it is terrible, lying there waiting for help to come. All come in awful condition, no previous care has been given to their wounds. It takes a lot of soaking to clean their wounds, dried blood, filth and dirt and lice. The bath house is not able to cope with the situation and neither can our limited staff and walking patients. Four of our nurses left for the Front, conditions are worse there. We do have a roof, a floor and everyone is fed after a fashion. No one works less than 12 hours in 24 and most of us do more. I see no one these days but my patients. I am happier than any time since in France, I feel I am really needed." *(July 29, 1918, Maude Frances Essig)*

"Battle casualties with open wounds required yet another plan of care in the preantibiotic era of World War I. Their treatment included extensive wound debridement and irrigation through perforated red rubber tubes with Carrel-Dakin solution (sodium hypochlorite) to deal with the inevitable infection. Staff administered tetanus antitoxin to all such patients routinely. Nurses cared for those with orthopaedic injuries in Bradford frames and extension devices for traction." *(Sarnecky, p. 96)*.

(Opposite) *Irrigation of patient wounds.*

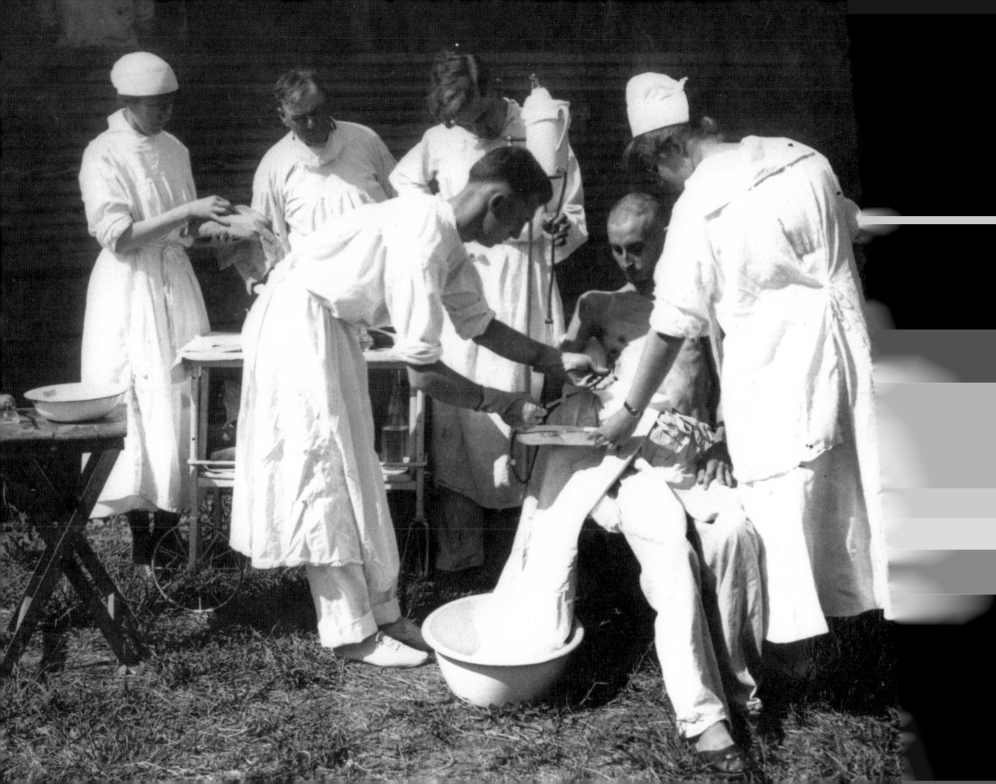

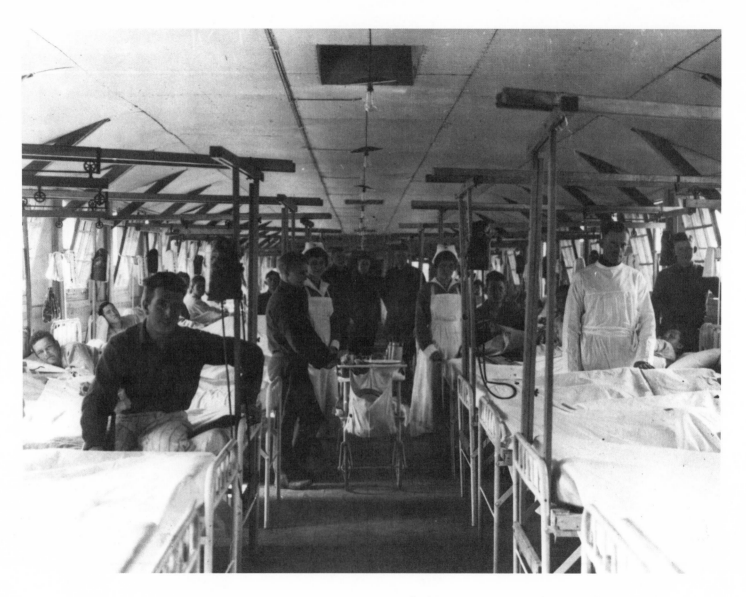

Ward of Evacuation Hospital No. 20 showing Balkan frames.

Hospital Trains

"HOSPITAL TRAINS FORMED THE CONNECTING LINK between the front-line and the base hospitals. Each train unit was complete, frequently organized as such in the United States; however, nurses were not attached to the hospital trains until several months after the hospital-train service had been functioning. The duties of the three nurses assigned to each of the trains were outlined in general instructions which were issued to the officers in charge of the trains:

> The senior of the three nurses assigned to the train will act as matron. Nurses will carry out the orders of the medical officers, and are to be obeyed next after them."

"The nurses were assigned quarters within the staff coach, and one of them was obliged always to be on duty. When it was possible for a nurse to leave, she could be gone no longer than two hours." *(The Medical Dept in the World War, Vol. XIII, p. 335)*

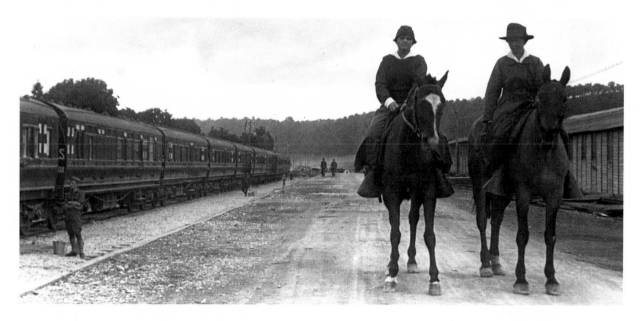

Mildred Brown and Ruth Lythe out for a ride, showing hospital train and Evacuation Hospital No. 8, Bazoilles, France, October 1918.

"The duties of the nurses on hospital trains were performed under difficulties. It was necessary for them to accustom themselves to the restricted quarters, the constant motion, and the uncertainty and irregularity of the hours of duty. The character of the duty on the hospital trains made it imperative that extreme care be exercised in the selection of nurses for such details. The limited space, the necessity for close association of officers and nurses, and the isolation from other groups of workers made hospital train duty a severe test of the persons assigned to it. Professional skill, great physical endurance, adaptability to unusual living and working conditions, ability to meet emergencies, and the possession of steadfast high principles were some of the qualifications found to be most desirable in a nurse on duty with a hospital train." *(The Medical Dept in the World War, Vol. XIII, p. 335)*

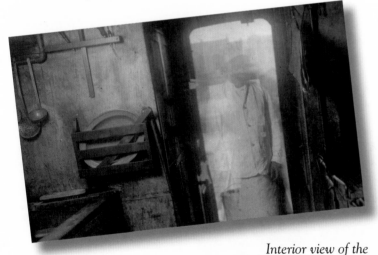

Interior view of the kitchen, where all meals for both the organization and patients were prepared. July 1919.

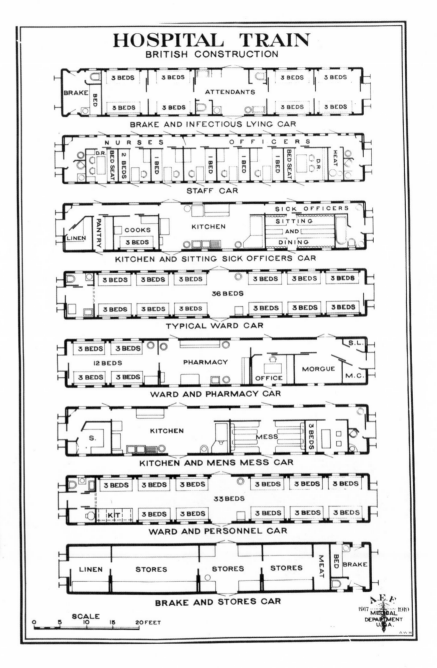

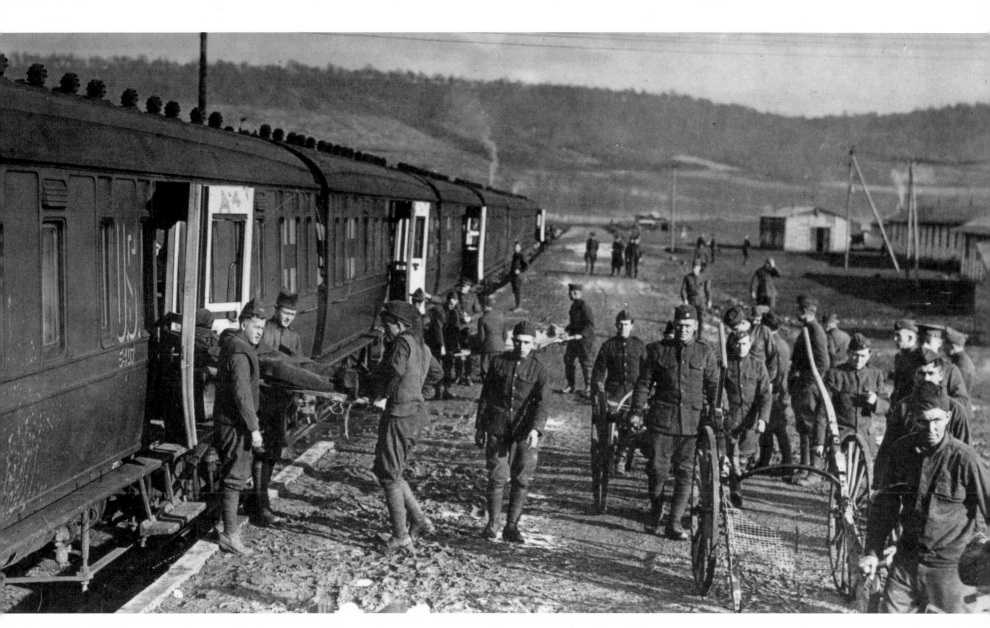

Soldiers loading evacuation train.

(Left) *Interior of a Glennon bunk car, Army hospital train, ready to receive the wounded from the transport. July 1919.*

(Opposite) *The interior of an Army hospital train showing the operating room, which may be used in case of medical emergency. July 1919.*

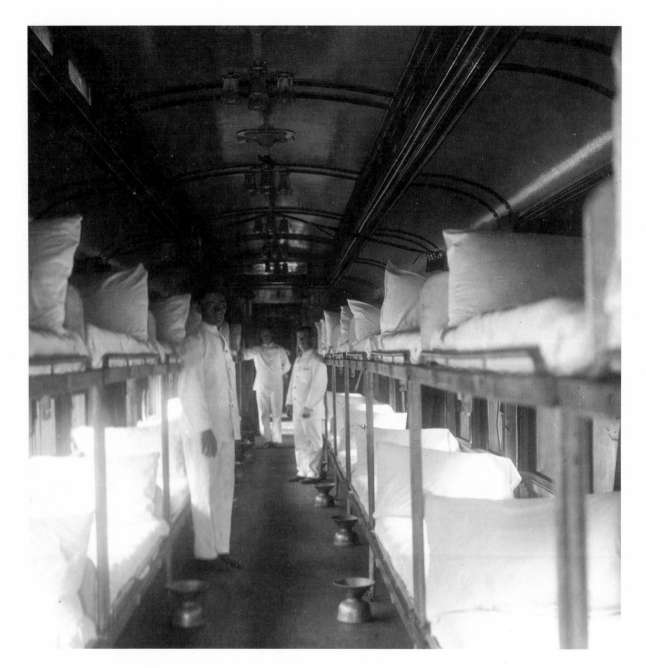

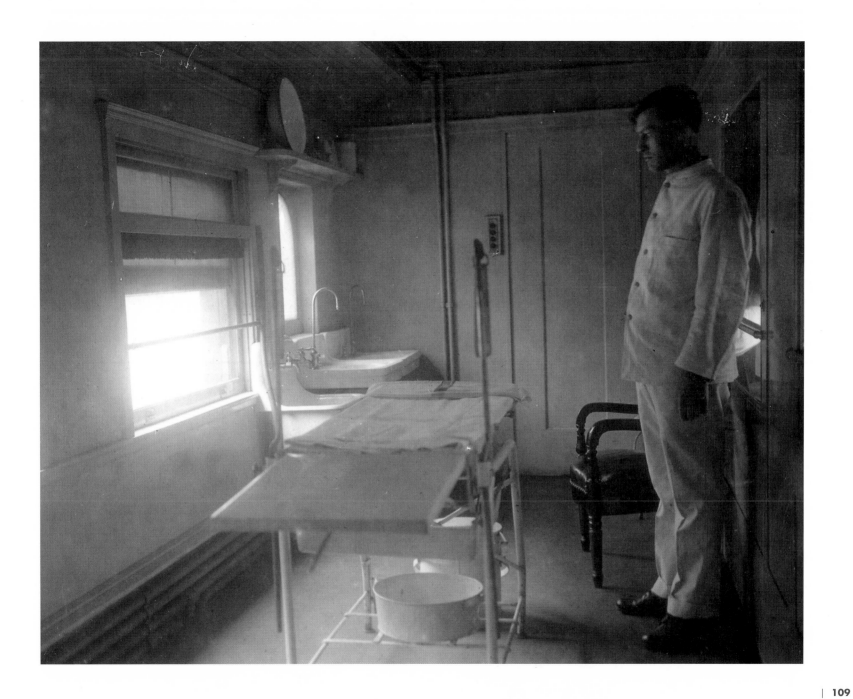

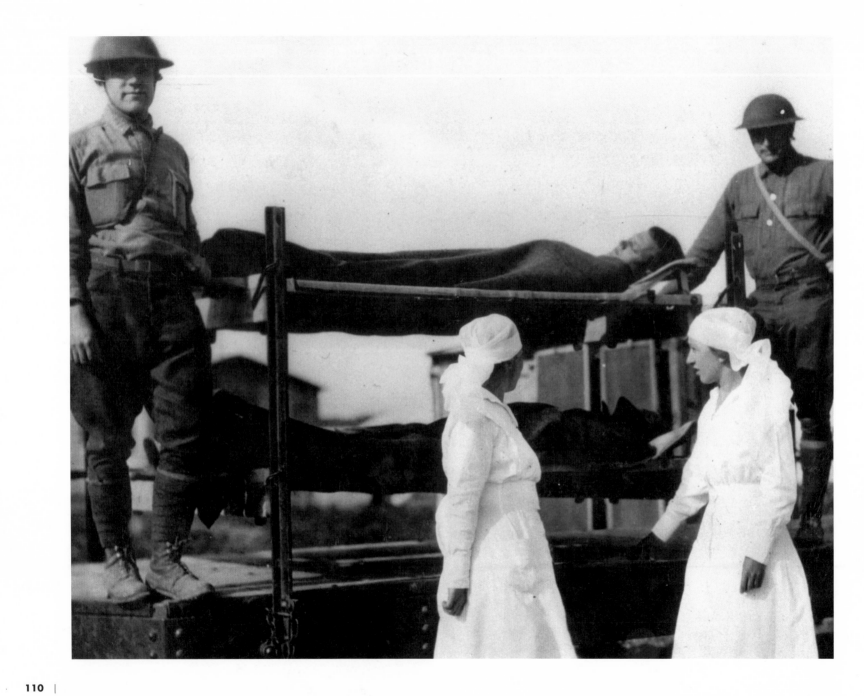

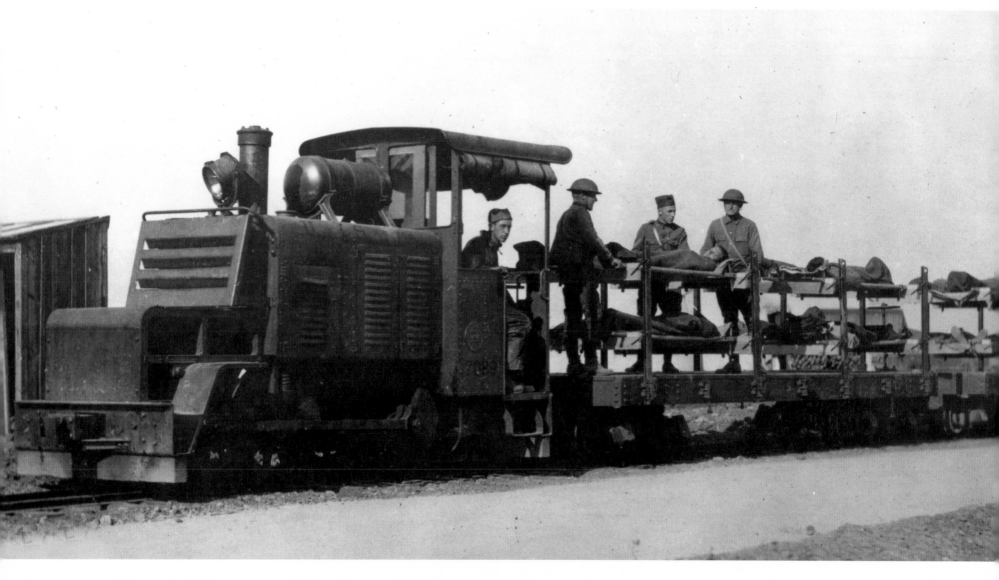

(Opposite) *Army nurses assess patients prior to evacuation on a hospital train.*

(Above) *Shunting engine with flat cars, used to evacuate wounded soldiers.*

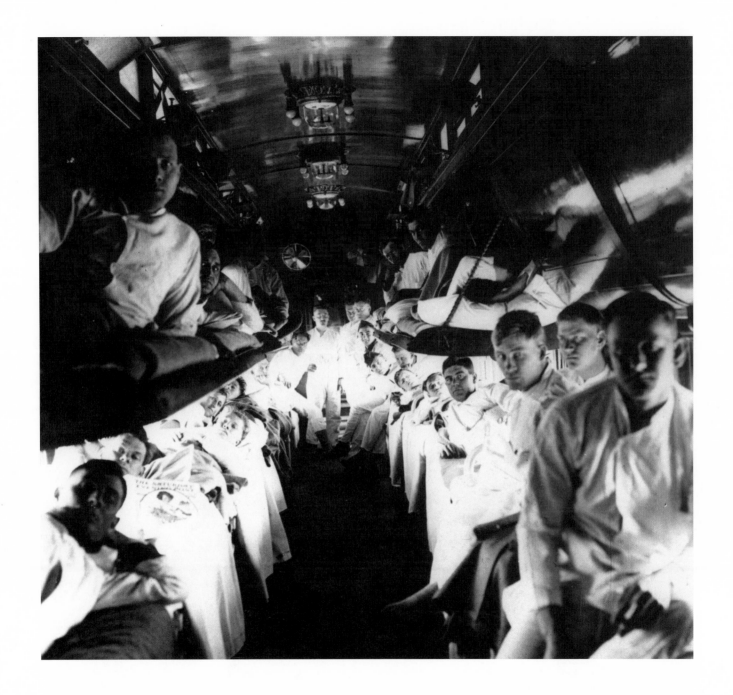

Camp Hospitals

"ARMY NURSES WERE ASSIGNED TO camp hospitals, which in most instances were in isolated areas but which functioned much in the same fashion as base hospitals, only on a smaller scale." *(The Medical Dept in the World War, Vol. XIII, p. 334)*

The following types of cases were treated from December 21, 1917, to about May 14, 1918: bronchitis, tonsillitis, influenza, and other acute minor illnesses, venereal cases, and minor surgical cases. *(Surgeon General Report, 1919, Vol. II, p. 2063)*

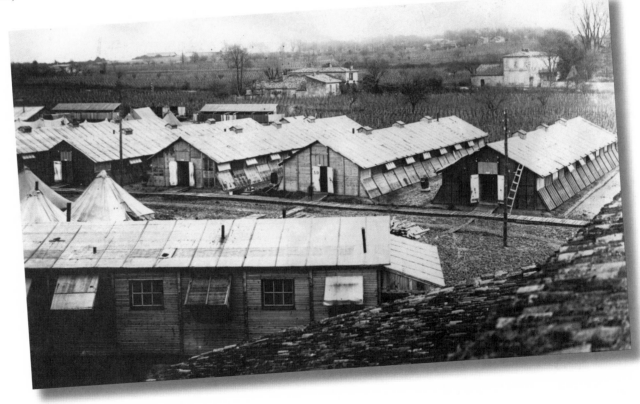

The first patients were admitted to Camp Hospital No. 2 at Bassens, France, on December 21, 1917. The hospital at this time consisted of two wards with 30 beds to each ward; one ward for white and one for black enlisted personnel.

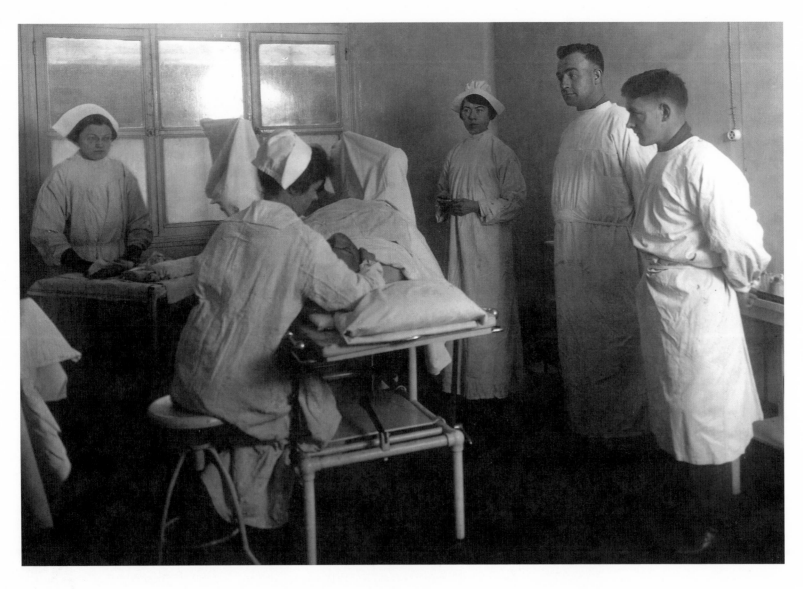

(Above) *Operating room functioning during an operation at Camp Hospital No. 27, Tours, France.*

(Opposite) *Early in September 1918, a venereal segregation camp was established as a part of Camp Hospital No. 15.*

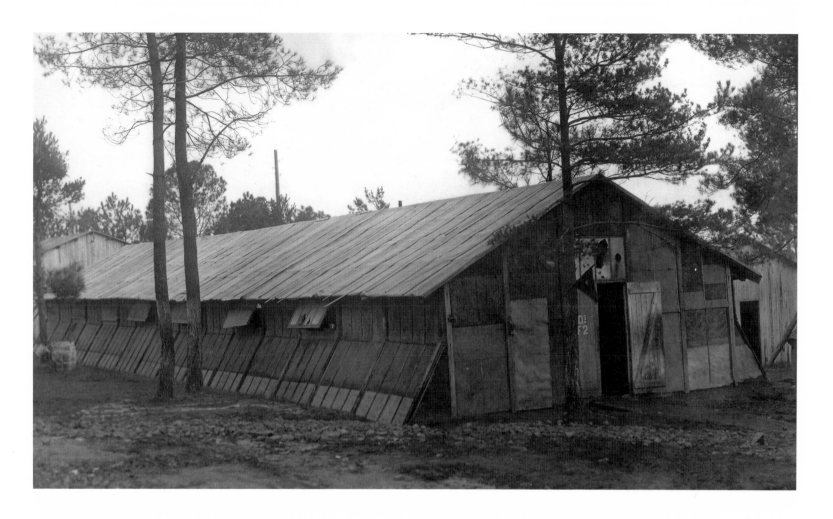

"Camp Hospital No. 15 was opened in October, 1917. It is part of Camp Coetquidan, an old artillery training camp taken over from the French. On November 1, 1917, when the hospital really commenced to receive patients, the personnel consisted of 1 medical officer, in addition to the commanding officer, and 37 enlisted men." *(Surgeon General Report, 1919, p. 2081)*

From December 1917 to January 1919, Florence A. Blanchfield was the acting chief nurse of Camp Hospital No. 15. By World War II Colonel Blanchfield served as Superintendent over all 56,000 Army nurses.

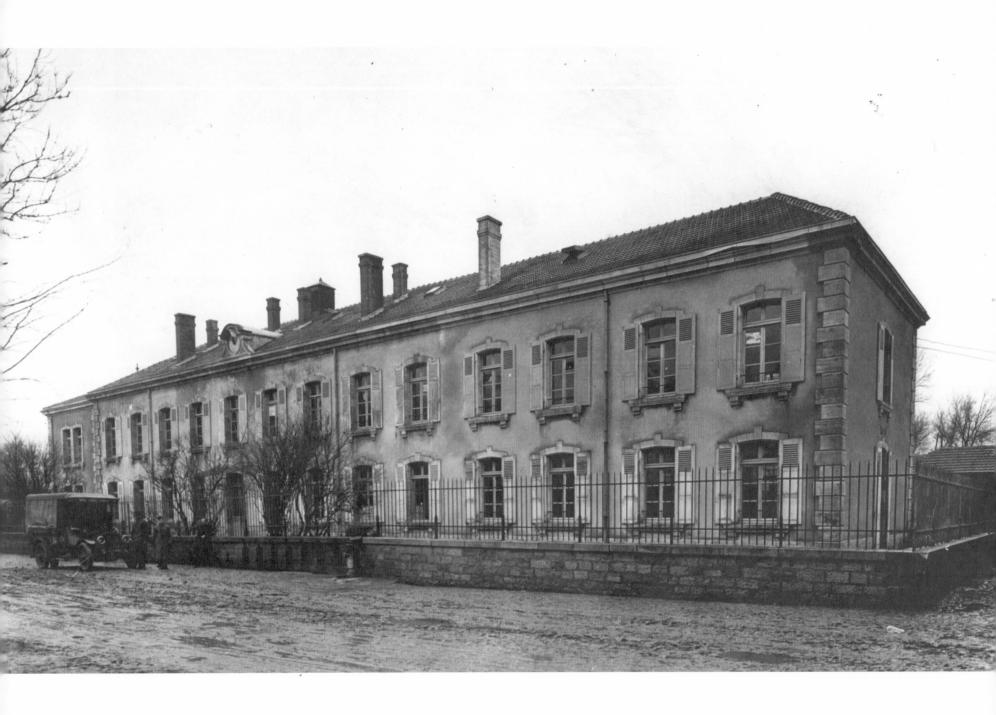

"Camp Hospital No. 22, situated at Langres (Haute-Marne), American Expeditionary Forces, was opened on or about November 15, 1917. The hospital was taken over January 5, 1918, with personnel consisting of a detachment from the 163rd Field Hospital. From January 5, 1918, to June 11, 1918, the hospital was operated on a basis of 100-bed capacity.

"This building is of stone, two stories and an unfinished third floor, used as a squad room for the enlisted personnel. A barrack or hut building was constructed in the rear as a kitchen and mess hall. The building was steam heated, and an electric lighting system was installed by the Engineer Corps and operated from the central station in the barracks. The water supply was originally from the French system, later supplemented by a pipe system, installed by the Americans, giving running tap water in the kitchen, operating room, washrooms, and toilets.

The general sanitation of the area was carried out by a sanitary squad, including the delousing of large numbers of troops coming through from the front. Only the sanitation of the building and grounds of the hospital was under the supervision of the hospital staff." *(Surgeon General Report, 1919, p. 2086)*

(Opposite) *Camp Hospital No. 22, situated at Langres, France.*

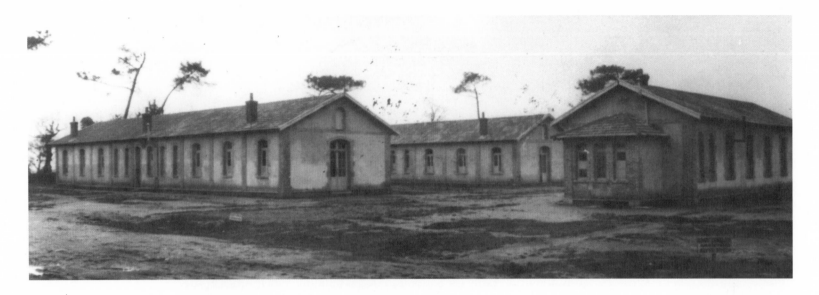

"Camp Hospital No. 31, *Camp de Meucon*, was situated on a narrow-guage railroad in the French Department of Morbihan, Brittany. This railroad connected the camp with the city of Vannes (12 kilometers away). The hospital occupies the site of what was formerly an old French artillery training camp, but was newly erected to serve the needs of an artillery training camp for the American Expeditionary Forces. The hospital site was about 3 kilometers from the AEF camp. The buildings that already existed on the old site were rebuilt and converted to suit the needs of the American hospital. They consisted of 12 low, stone buildings, of barracks type construction and various smaller buildings of wood and stone. The 12 buildings referred to are now being used as wards and have a capacity of 60 beds each.

A new surgical building of brick and stone houses the pharmacy, dental office, eye, ear, nose and throat clinic, pathological lab and X-ray room." *(Surgeon General Report, 1919, p. 2097)*

(Above) *Nurses quarters at Camp Hospital No. 31.*

(Opposite) *X-Ray Room, Camp Hospital No. 31, Morbihan, Brittany.*

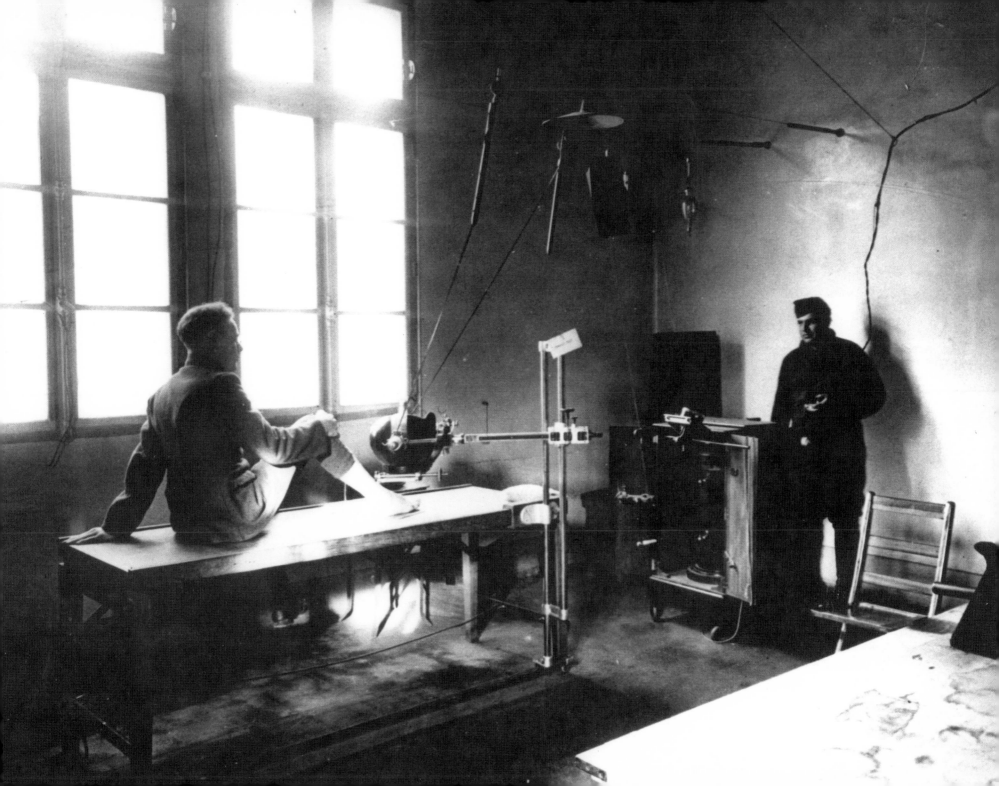

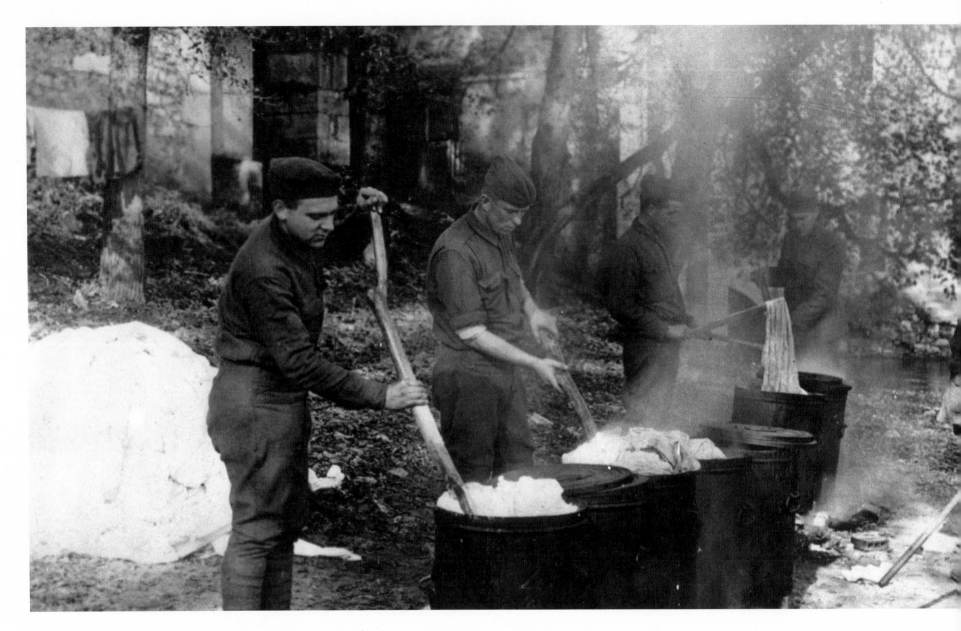

Sterilizing laundry at Camp Hospital No. 78, 84th Division, Chateau La Roche (Dordogne, France), November 4, 1918.

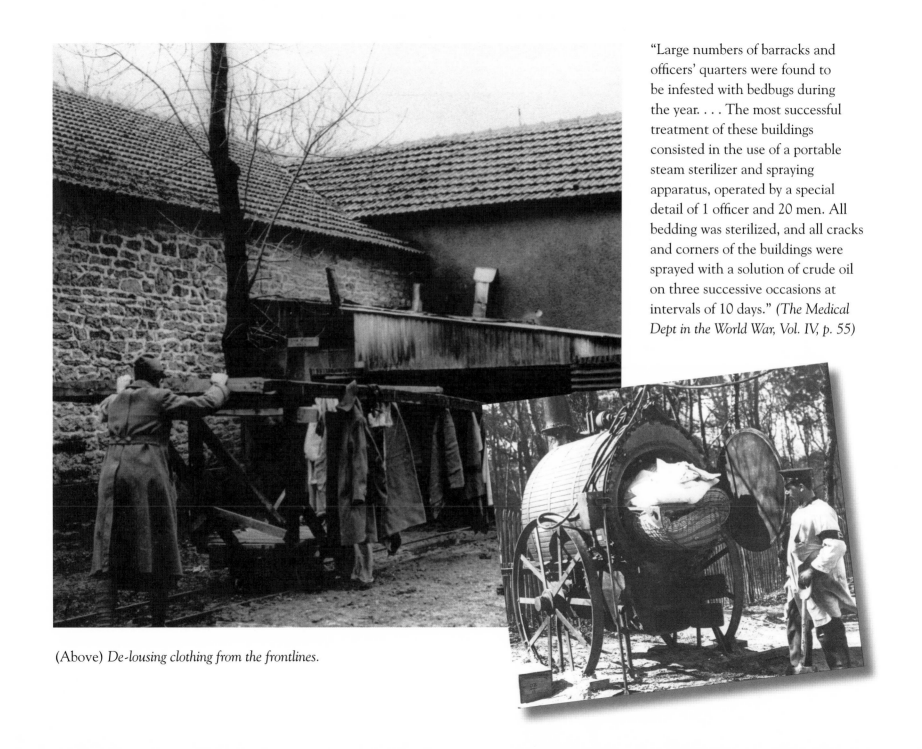

"Large numbers of barracks and officers' quarters were found to be infested with bedbugs during the year. . . . The most successful treatment of these buildings consisted in the use of a portable steam sterilizer and spraying apparatus, operated by a special detail of 1 officer and 20 men. All bedding was sterilized, and all cracks and corners of the buildings were sprayed with a solution of crude oil on three successive occasions at intervals of 10 days." *(The Medical Dept in the World War, Vol. IV, p. 55)*

(Above) *De-lousing clothing from the frontlines.*

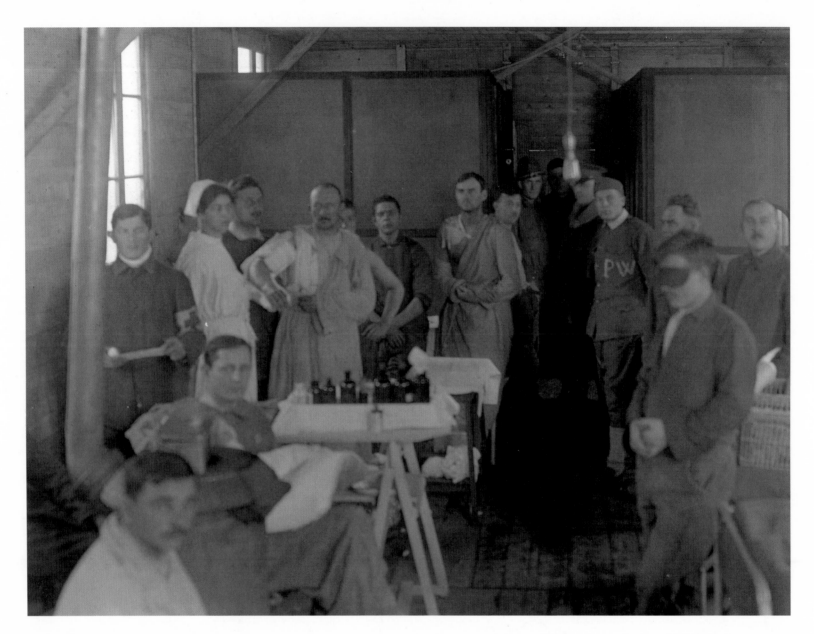

(Both views) *German prisoner ward, Camp Hospital No. 27, Tours, France.*

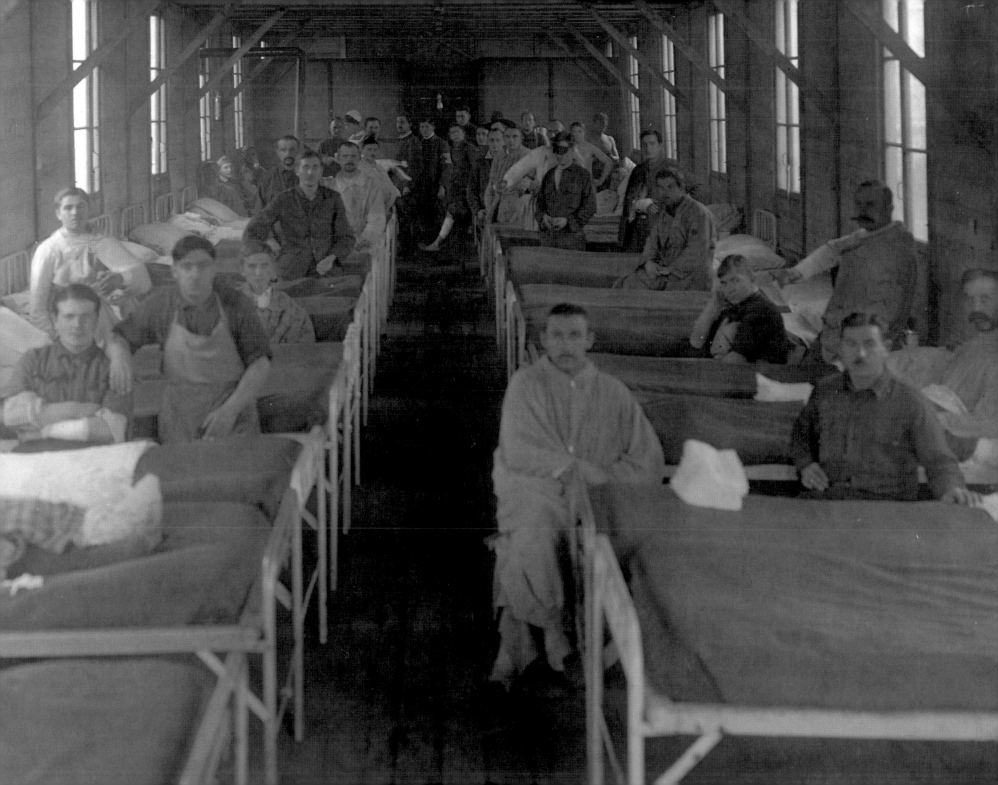

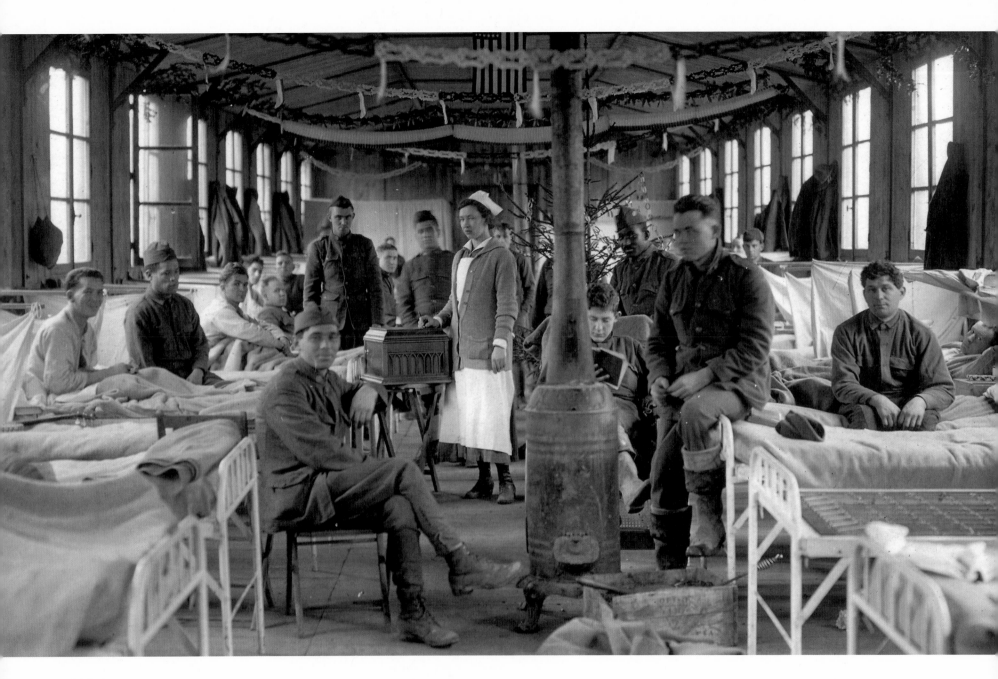

"Camp Hospital No. 68 is situated in a portion of the College de Jeunes Filles, No. 10 rue Littre, Bourges, Department of Cher. The portion used by the Americans is located at the rear of the court—3-story stone building, with roomy basement and a spacious, well-ventilated attic. In this building is located the hospital proper.

This hospital was established with one thought ever foremost, i.e., not to make it the largest in the American Expeditionary [F]orces, but to make it the best. To have the lowest death rate and the least suffering was the constant aim of every man and woman. The building was formally turned over to the Americans on October 1.

On December 1 the hospital was averaging about 150 patients, and every increase in bed capacity only met the demands. The necessity for increased room made it necessary to procure and erect five tents in the courtyard, bringing the total number of beds to 180." (*Surgeon General Report, 1919, p. 2127*)

(Opposite) *A festive ward 12 (medical), Camp Hospital No. 33, Brest, Finistere, France, December 1918.*

(Right) *Camp Hospital; No. 68, College de Jeunes Filles, No. 10 rue Littre, Bourges, France.*

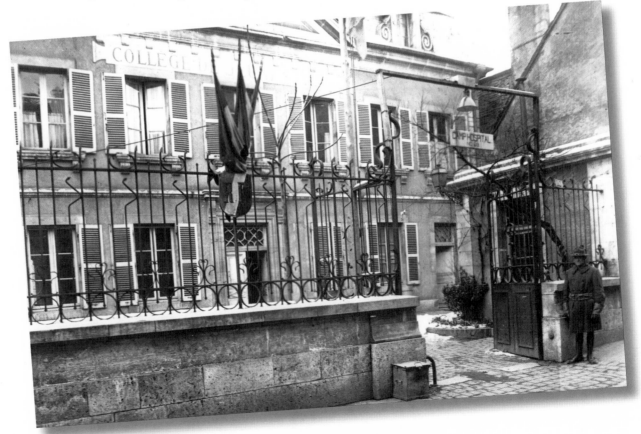

Behind the Lines

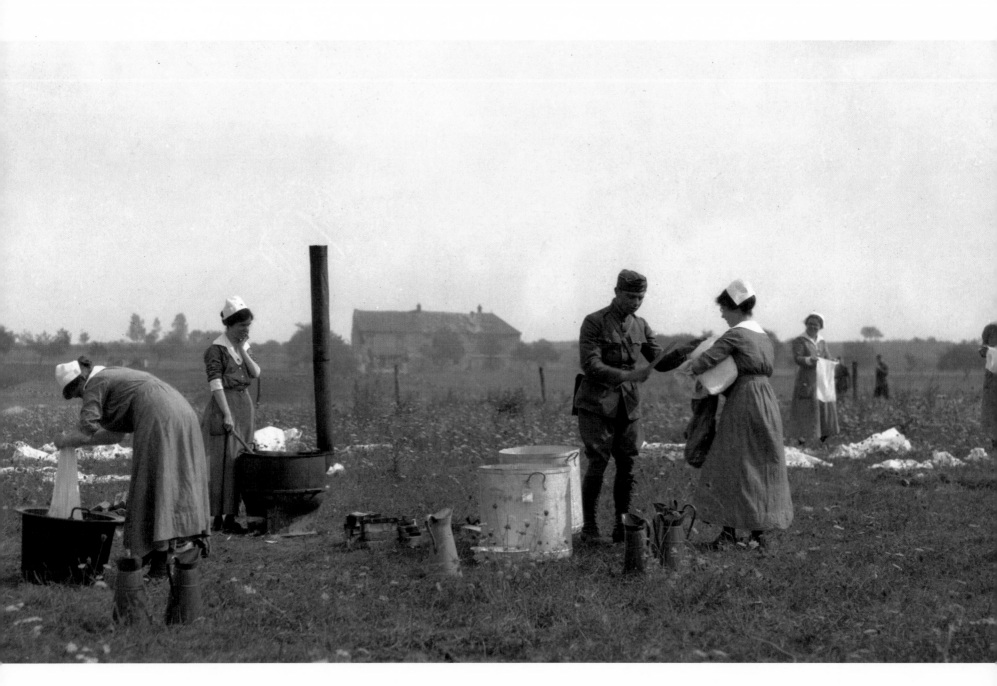

Quarters and Living Conditions

"FOR THE NURSES THE QUESTION OF LAUNDRY led to much discomfort. Some of the hospitals were able to provide their own laundries, some secured French women to do the work, and sometimes the work was done in French laundries in neighboring towns. In many cases, however, the nurses themselves had to launder their own clothing, including their uniforms. This was a hardship, particularly during the times when their physical strength was taxed to the utmost in caring for their patients. The director of nursing service on her inspections of nurses' quarters noted but few rooms in which during the winter months, flannels were not hanging to dry. The lack of proper facilities for laundry work and the dampness of the winter months made it necessary for many of the nurses' rooms to be 'festooned' with wet flannels from one week end to another. Mobile hospitals which were equipped with portable laundries seemed to solve the problem in the best way." *(The Medical Dept in the World War, Vol. XIII, p. 338)*

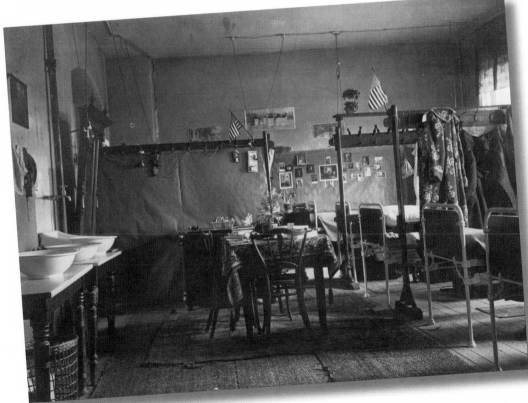

Nurses' bedroom and dining area at Camp Hospital No. 24, Langres, France.

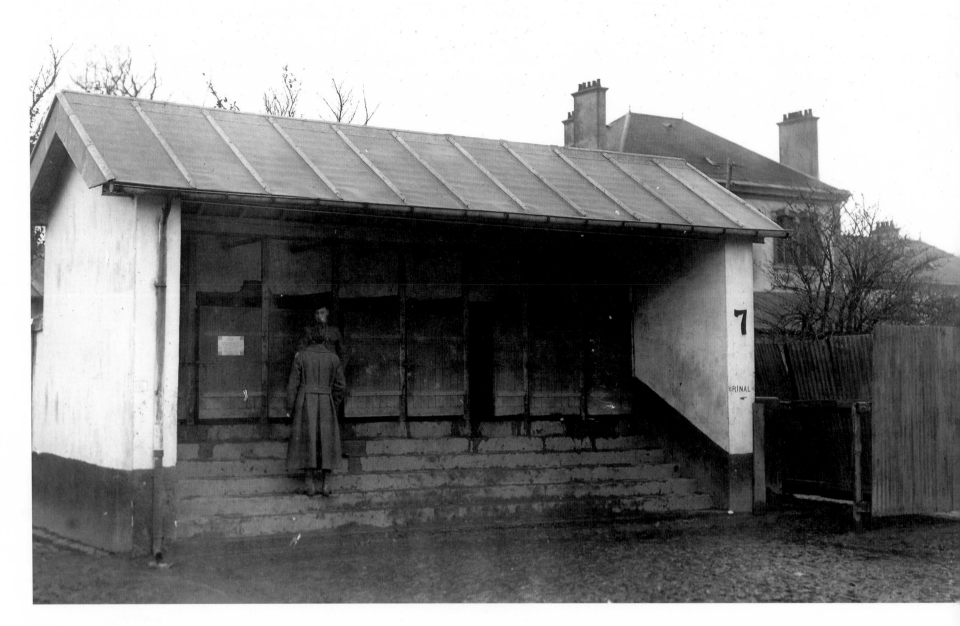

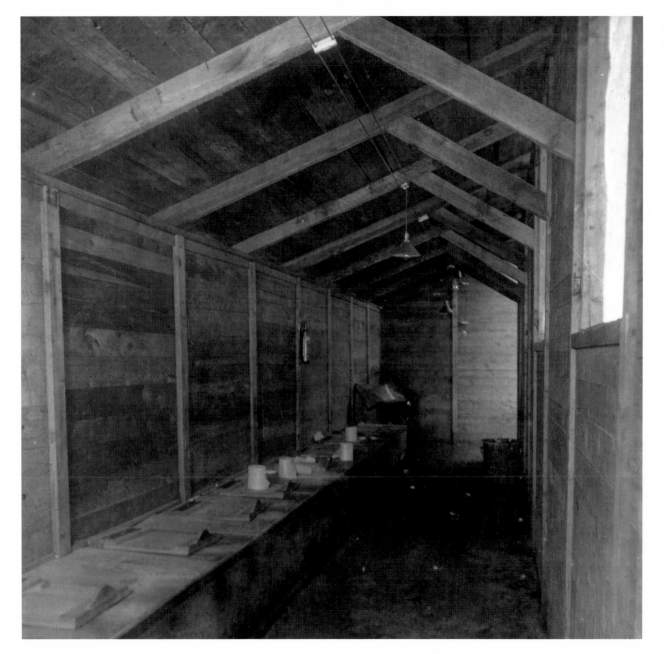

Latrine views at Camp Hospital No. 33, Brest, France.

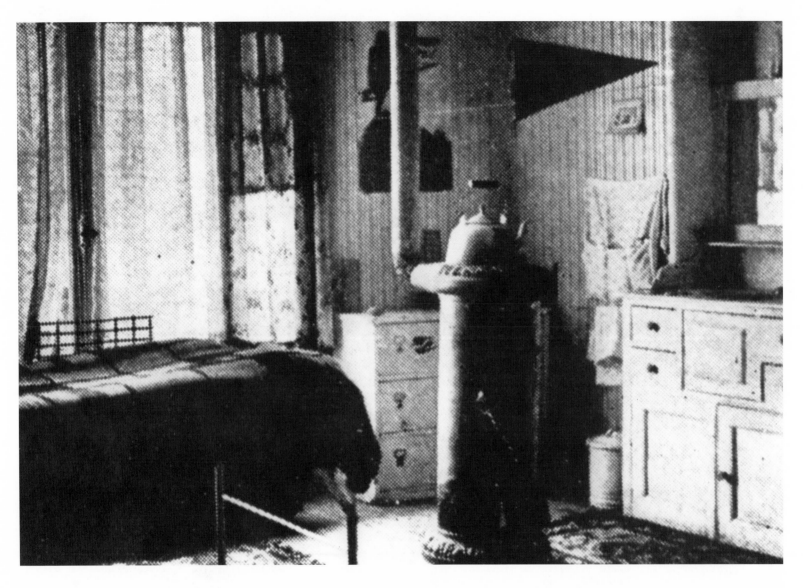

(Above) *Nurses' quarters at Base Hospital No. 20, Chatel Guyon, France.*

(Opposite) *Interior of nurses' quarters of the "semi-permanent" barracks type.*

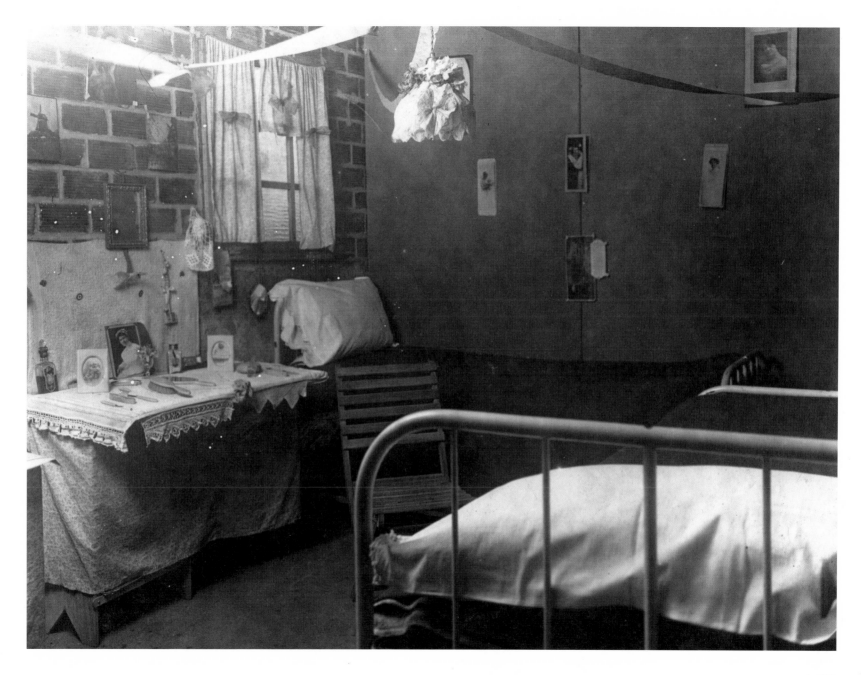

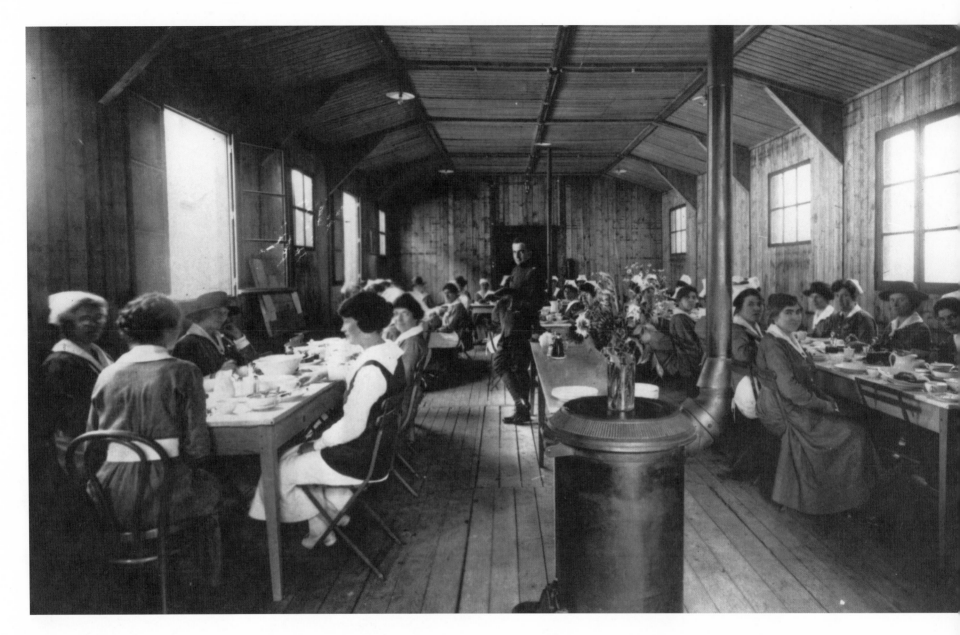

Nurses' mess hall at Base Hospital No. 17 in Dijon, France, September 5, 1918.

Leisure

REST, RELAXATION, AND RECREATION were important to Army nurses whether they were in France, England, or back in the United States. Yet in France, "opportunities for recreation for nurses were often very limited. Muddy roads frequently eliminated walking in places where that was the only chance for diversion. Dim lights prevented reading, writing, or sewing in the nurses' rooms, and even when general living rooms were provided they frequently were too cold and too poorly lighted to permit of any enjoyment from playing cards or other indoor games. In the hospital centers the American Red Cross gradually provided recreation huts equipped with libraries, moving-picture apparatus, and musical instruments; in some places they even built special huts for the nurses' recreation houses. These recreation houses were like private clubhouses and were fitted with assembly rooms, libraries, kitchens, sewing rooms, and laundries." *(The Medical Dept in the World War, Vol. XIII, pp. 338–339)*

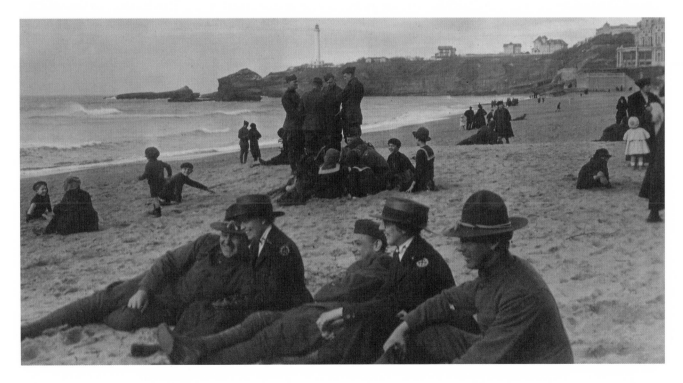

Sunday afternoon on the beach at a popular leave area in Biarritz, France.

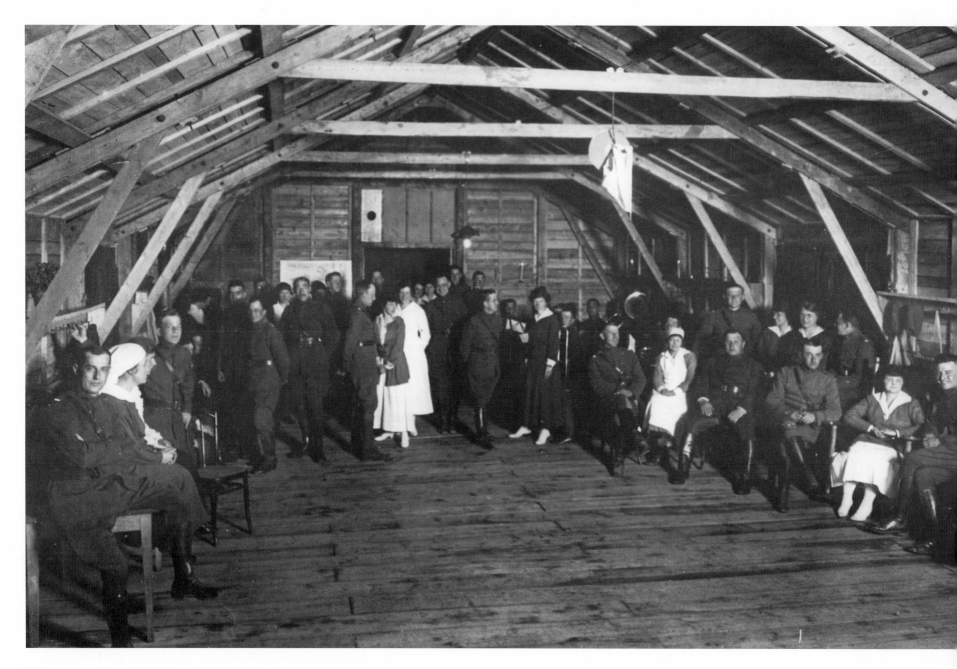

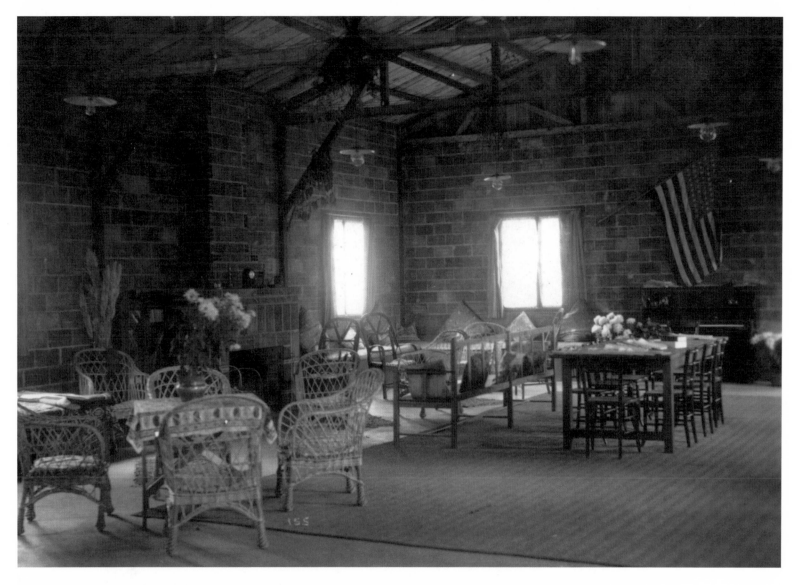

(Opposite) *Evening dance for the staff of Evacuation Hospital No. 1 (26th Division), on May 7, 1918, at Sebastopol, France.*

(Above) *The nurses' recreation hut at Angers, France.*

(Right) *"Pride" was played by Mary Devine, a nurse at Base Hospital No. 101, in this patriotic play.*

(Opposite) *A cast of nurses, officers, and enlisted men who took part in "Democracy Victorious" at Base Hospital No. 101, St. Nazaire, on July 4, 1918.*

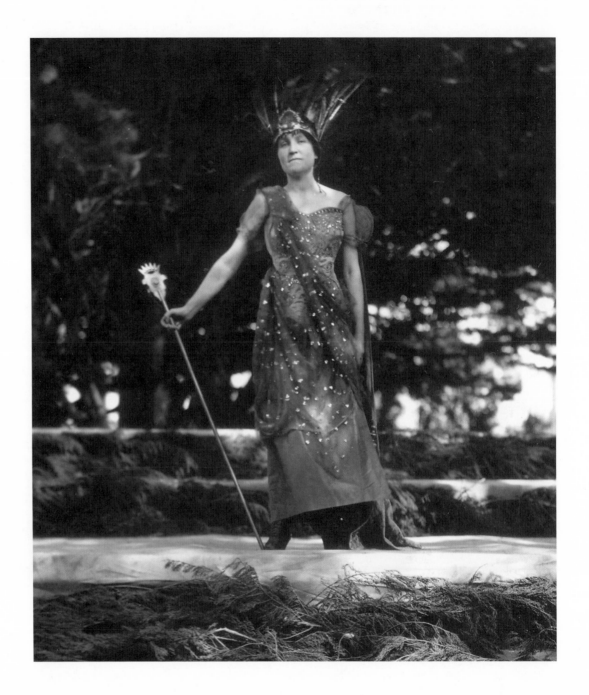

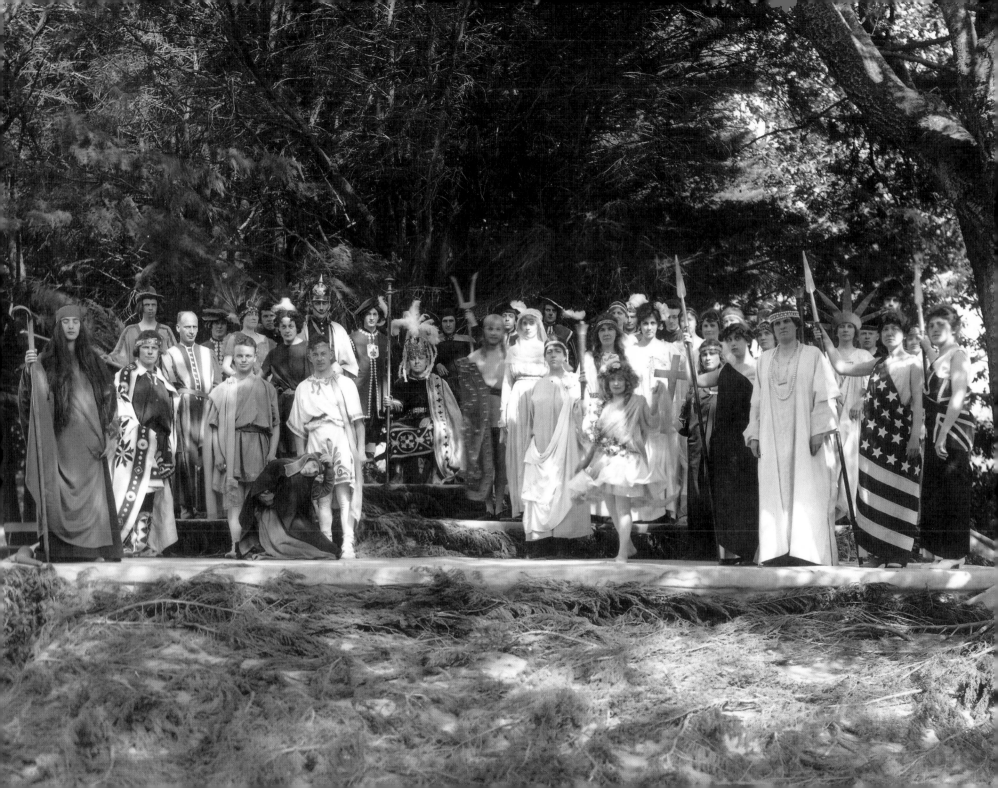

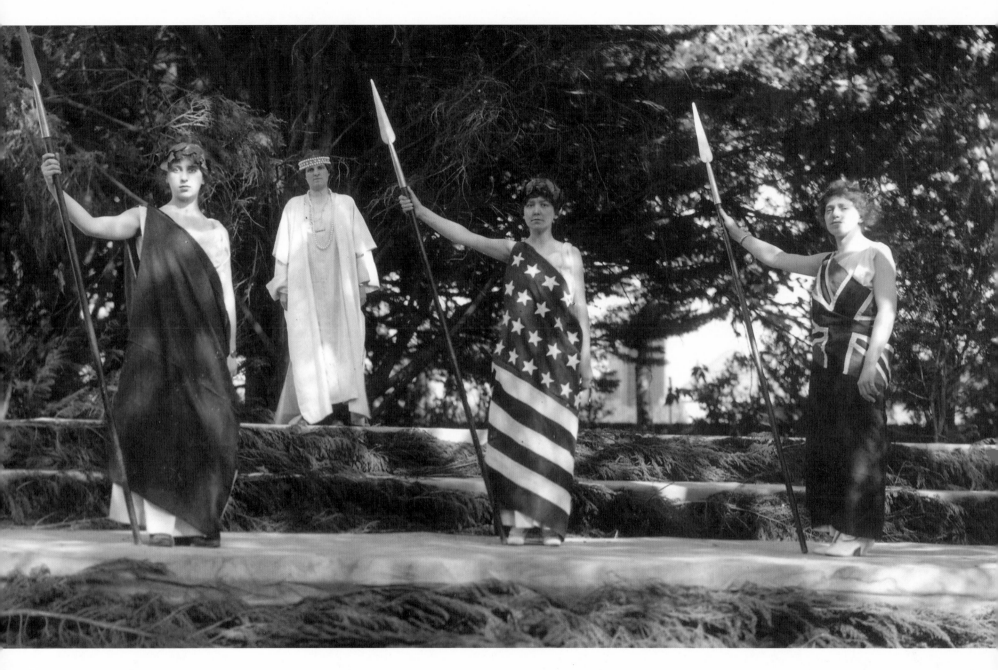

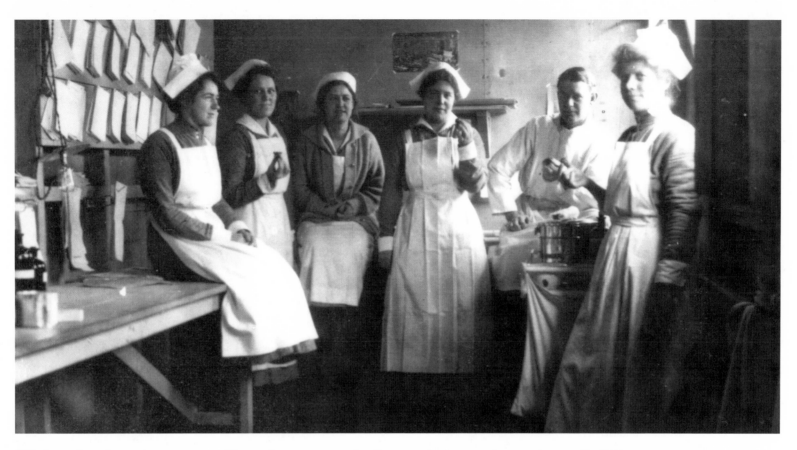

"We have found a way to get sugar. We can buy two pounds of sugar at a time, each one of us, at the U.S. commissary and we got some cocoa [at] a French store and also got some walnuts. We made fudge a couple of nights ago. I tell you it did taste good. The first fudge we have had a chance to make. We are going to enjoy life a little more now." *(December 12, 1918, Elizabeth Lewis, Vichy, France)*

(Above) *A popular pastime—fudgemaking party on the ward at Base Hospital No. 34. Participants and date unknown.*

(Opposite) *"The Allies" featuring Nurse Beaumont as France, Nurse Woeckner as America, and Nurse Randall as Great Britain. In the rear is "Democracy," a role played by Nurse Morriss.*

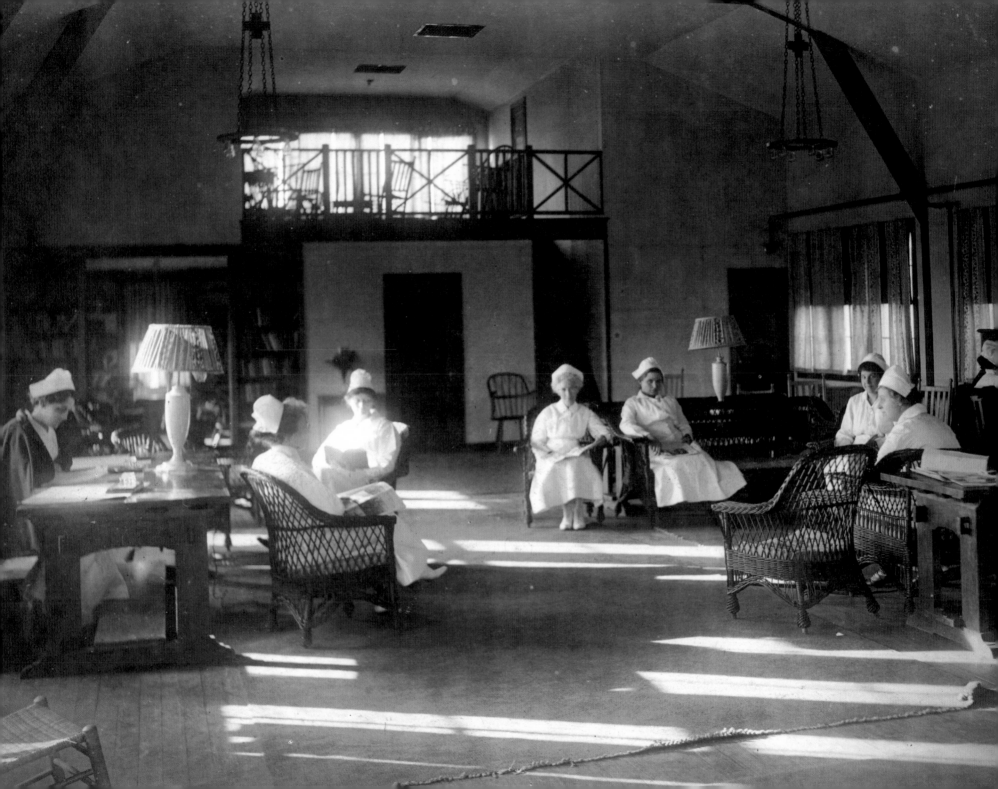

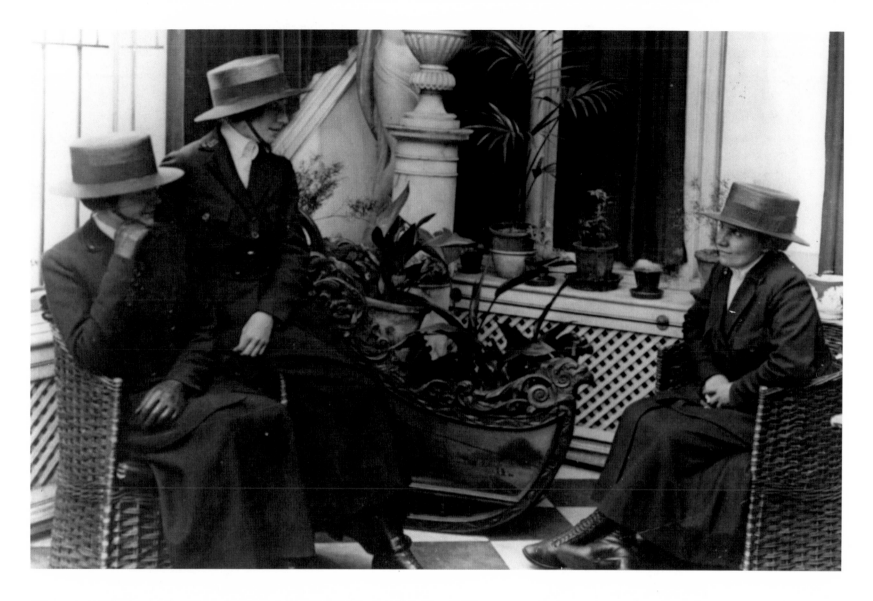

(Opposite) *Relaxing in the Nurses Recreation Hut in Washington, DC (Fox Hills).*

(Above) *American Red Cross Nurses' Club in London, England.*

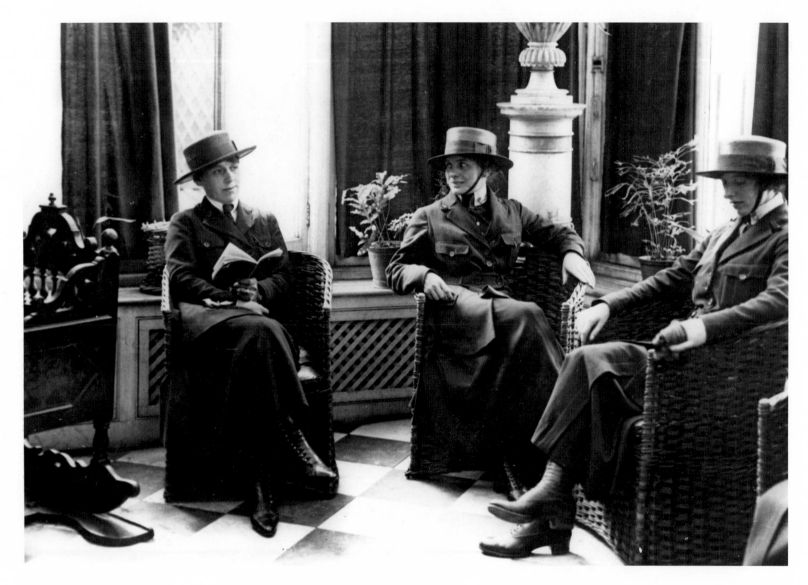

(Above) *Relaxing in the Conservatory of the ARC Nurses Club in London, England.*

(Opposite) *Nurses wearing straw blue hats authorized for summer wear.*

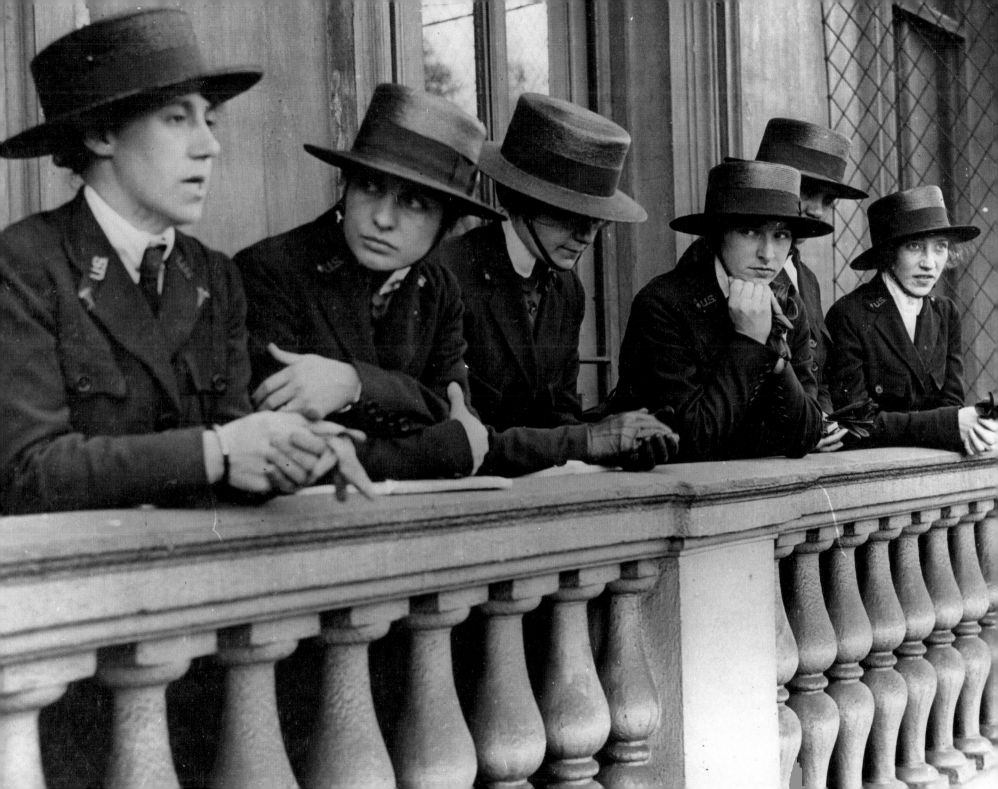

"In February, 1918, the United States Army established a leave-area center in Aix-les-Bains, Savoie, France. This proved such a success that soon other parts [of the provinces] were secured and turned into an Alpine playground for the American Expeditionary Forces. . . . The real purpose of a leave area is to give health and happiness to the Army and so increase the vigor and efficiency of the whole American Expeditionary Forces. In this work the hospital plays a very important role, not only in caring for those already ill, but also by establishing dispensaries and inaugurating methods of sanitation for the prevention of disease." (*Surgeon General Report, 1919, p. 2116*)

(Opposite) *The Grand Hôtel Beau-Site, Aix-les-Bains, France.*

The following are views from an advertising brochure for the Grand Hôtel Beau-Site in Aix-les-Bains, France, dated January 1919.

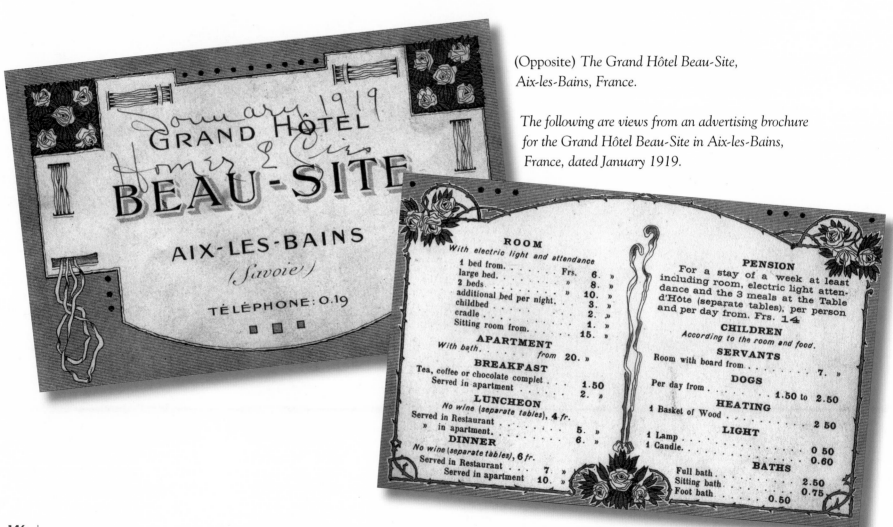

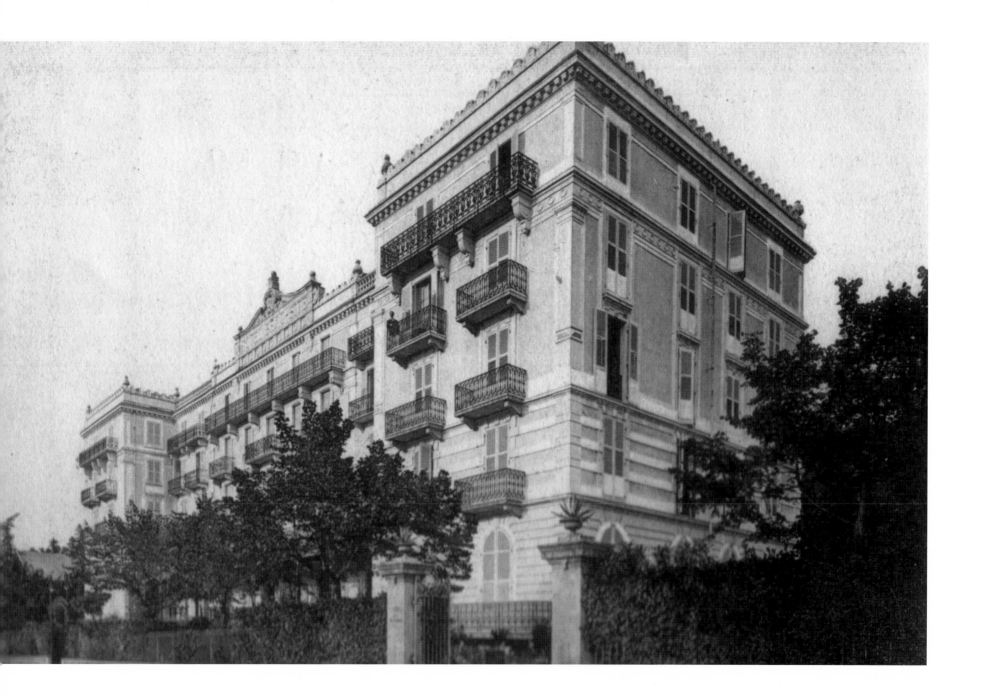

"Aug. [?] [1918] Saturday—we arrived at Aix-les-Bains at 7:30 AM. Signed in with the A.P.M. [Assistant Provost Marshall]. Breakfasted at the Depot, then searched for rooms. With a lot of persuasion and $1.00 we were given accommodations at Thermal Establishment Hotel. We waited for ages for a room, so went across the street to a wonderful Bath Establishment and had a wonderful bath. We were told J. Pierpont Morgan had a private suite here. It was all very grand and old, after lunch at the Hotel we crawled into our wonderful beds, box springs, feather mattress, and down quilt, and slept until Sunday morning. We were never so tired as when we retired and such luxury!" *(Maude Frances Essig, 1918)*

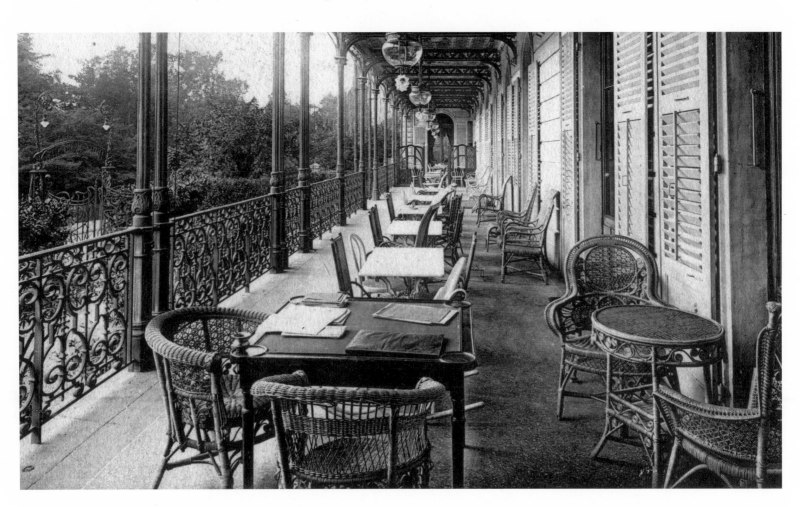

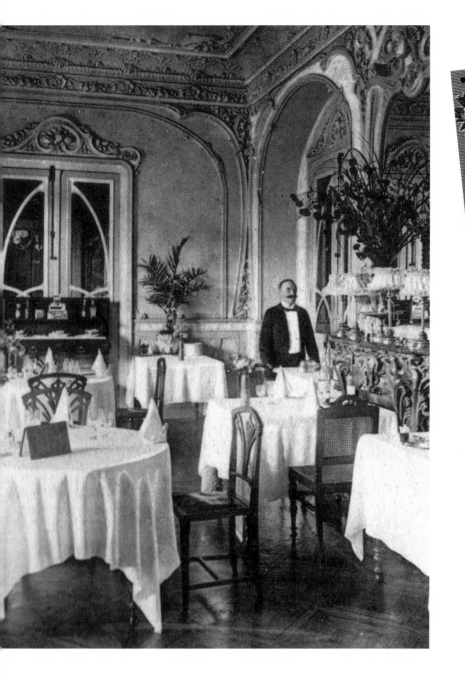

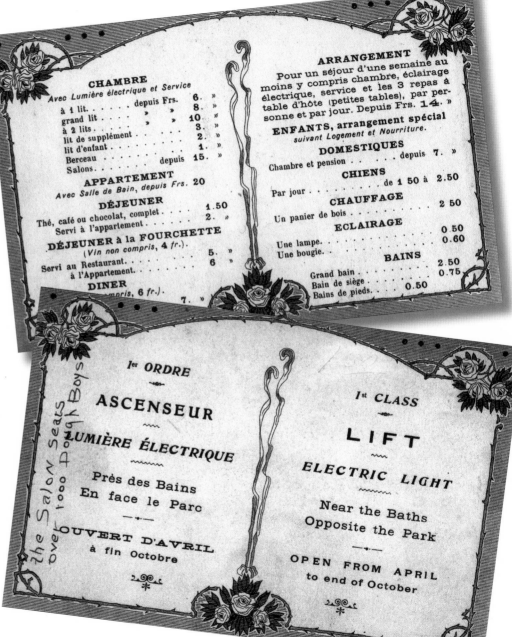

CHAMBRE

Avec Lumière électrique et Service

à 1 lit	depuis Frs.	6.
grand lit	»	8.
à 2 lits	»	10.
lit de supplément		3.
lit d'enfant		2.
Berceau		1.
Salons	depuis	15.

APPARTEMENT

Avec Salle de Bain, depuis Frs. 20

DÉJEUNER

Thé, café ou chocolat, complet	1.50
Servi à l'appartement	2.

DÉJEUNER à la FOURCHETTE

(Vin non compris, 4 fr.)

Servi au Restaurant	5.
à l'Appartement	6.

DINER

...mpris, 6 fr.)

7.

ARRANGEMENT

Pour un séjour d'une semaine au moins y compris chambre, éclairage électrique, service et les 3 repas à table d'hôte (petites tables), par personne et par jour. Depuis Frs. **14**.

ENFANTS, arrangement spécial

suivant Logement et Nourriture.

DOMESTIQUES

Chambre et pension	depuis	7.

CHIENS

Par jour	de 1 50 à 2.50

CHAUFFAGE

Un panier de bois	2 50

ECLAIRAGE

Une lampe	0.50
Une bougie	0.60

BAINS

	2.50
Grand bain	0.75
Bain de siège	
Bains de pieds	0.50

1er ORDRE

ASCENSEUR

LUMIÈRE ÉLECTRIQUE

Près des Bains
En face le Parc

OUVERT D'AVRIL
à fin Octobre

1st CLASS

LIFT

ELECTRIC LIGHT

Near the Baths
Opposite the Park

OPEN FROM APRIL
to end of October

The Salon Sears over 1000 Dough Boys

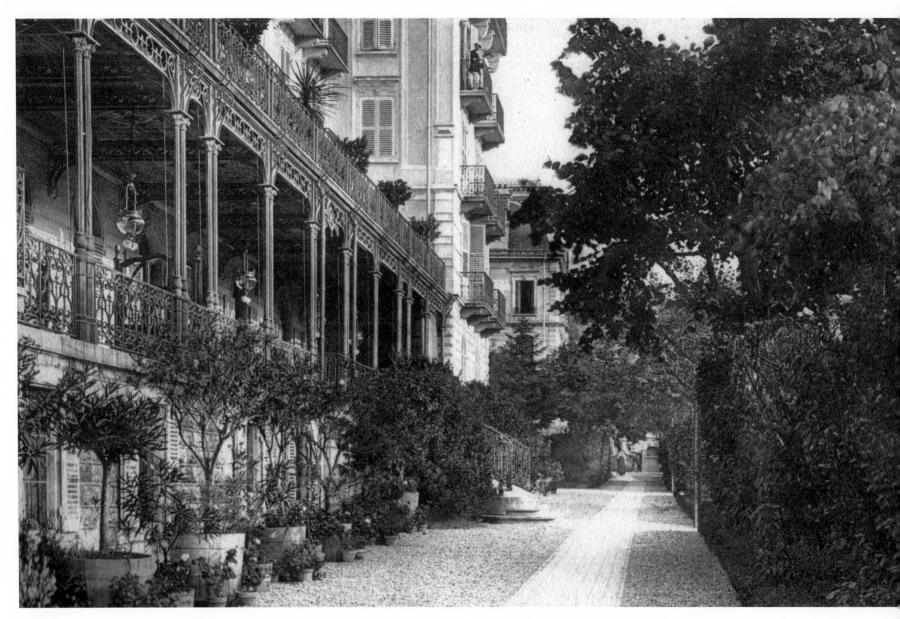

A rear view of The Grand Hôtel Beau-Site.

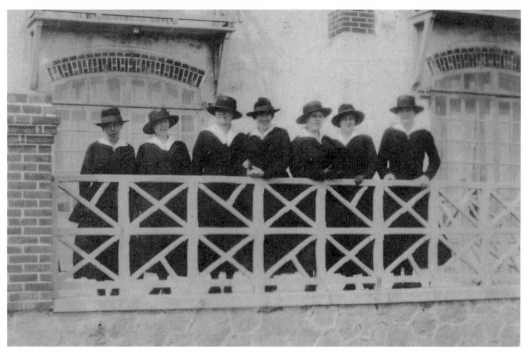

Quiberon, a commune of the French Department Morbihan, situated on a peninsula in the region of Brittany, is known as a seaside resort for the French during the summer and for its history of sardine production.

(Left) *Shown here are American nurses most likely stationed at a nearby camp hospital, enjoying the life of this beautiful area, outside a local villa.*

(Bottom) *Nurses on the beach at Quiberon, and with their housekeeper and her children.*

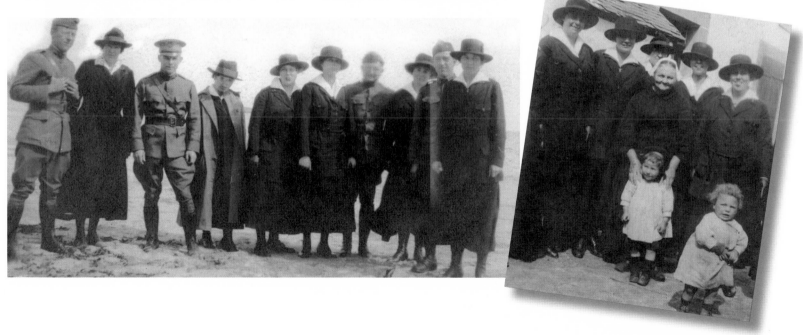

In the Operating Room

"A STEADY STREAM OF PATIENTS is carried into the X-ray room and from there either directly to the operating room or back to their tents. The plates are developed almost immediately and are examined while wet and stuck up in improvised holders on the windows of the operating room. They all showed foreign bodies and often bubbles, indicating the dreaded infection by the 'gas bacillus,' which causes such dreadful gas gangrene. All these cases have to be opened up and the necrotic tissue cleaned out. The supervisors were each on their side of the hospital, and the nurses were all getting the poor creatures as comfortable as possible. . . . Then we began in the operating room, taking out foreign bodies and incising and draining.

We took pieces of shell out of necks, hips, knees, skulls, ankles, shoulders, and out of the spine of my poor paralyzed man. Some of the men took the ether badly and screamed and fought and cursed; some thought they were in the battle and called out to their comrades." *(September 28, 1917, Stimson, Finding Themselves)*

(Left) *Triage at Base Hospital No. 45, Tours.*

(Opposite) *The G.U. (Genito-urinary) operating room at Base Hospital No. 57, Paris.*

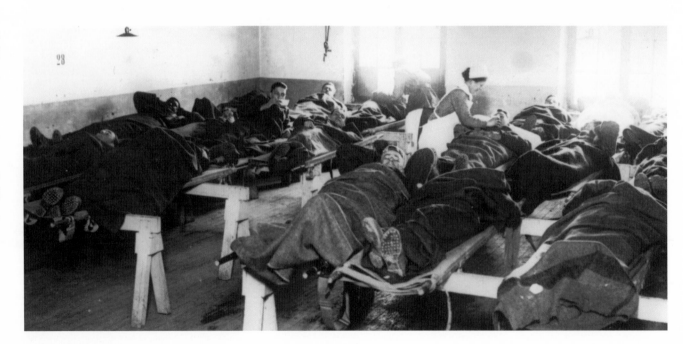

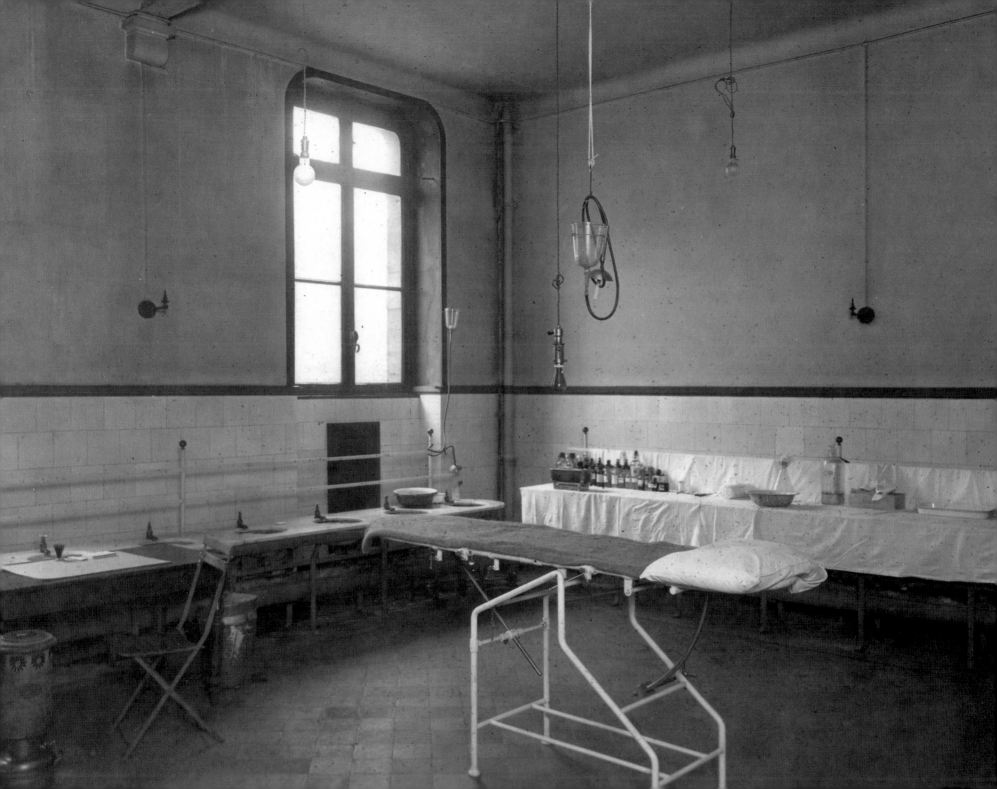

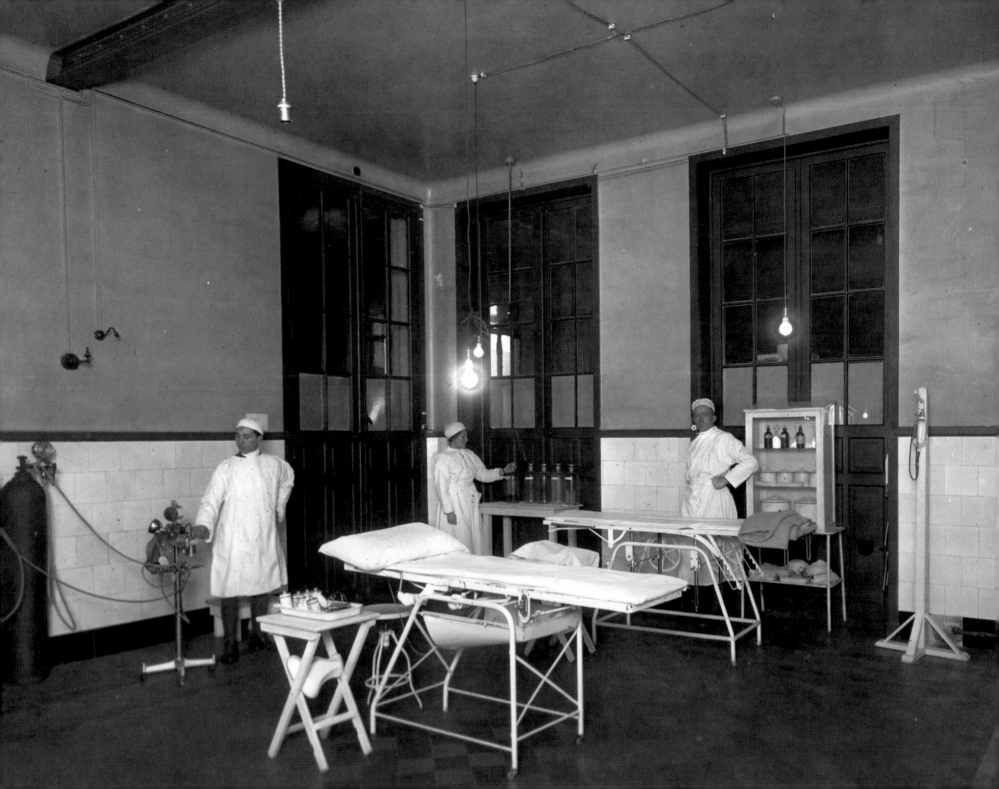

Base Hospital No. 57 took over a large school building and functioned as a part of the Paris district. The normal bed capacity of the hospital was 1,800, distributed in 75 wards, but during October 1918, as many as 2,000 sick and wounded were in the hospital. This hospital admitted both surgical and medical cases; the total number admitted during the war was 8,505. The hospital also operated a central dental infirmary, which cared for a majority of the dental cases in the district of Paris; 7,292 such patients received treatment during its period of activity.

Base Hospital No. 57 sailed from Brest, France, on August 13, 1919, aboard the *Kaiserine Augusta Victoria*, arrived in the United States on August 22, and was demobilized shortly afterward.

(Opposite) *Operating room. Private Nicholas Romeo, Alice Cahn, and Sergeant H.T. Aardweg, all listed on the Signal Corps photograph caption as "surgical assistants." U.S. Military Hospital No. 57, Medical Corps, Paris.*

"Early in the year 1917 the 1st Division was assembled in the United States ready for duty overseas, or wherever the United States needed Regular Army men. In June, 1917, they embarked for France, landing in St. Nazaire, and from its personnel of men and officers came the first patients to Base Hospital No. 101.

"On the 5th of June, 1917, some 37 nurses—members of the Nurse Reserve Corps—assembled in New York City. They came from many states in the union. They were soon attached to Base Hospital Unit 18, composed in the main of Johns Hopkins men.

"Embarking at New York on the *Finland* they landed in France on June 28 and went immediately to Savenay. After a few days they were ordered to St. Nazaire to join forces with the medical officers and medical department soldiers who had reached St. Nazaire at about the same time. The latter, numbering about 14 soldiers were ordered to make up the personnel of the hospital. Not having any official designation, the officers and men voted to call the hospital 'No. 1,' later the name being officially changed to United States Army Hospital No. 1." *(Surgeon General Report, 1919, p. 2004)*

(Opposite) Operations on shrapnel wounds in the operating room, Base Hospital No. 6, 26th Division, Sebastopol, France, May 2, 1918.

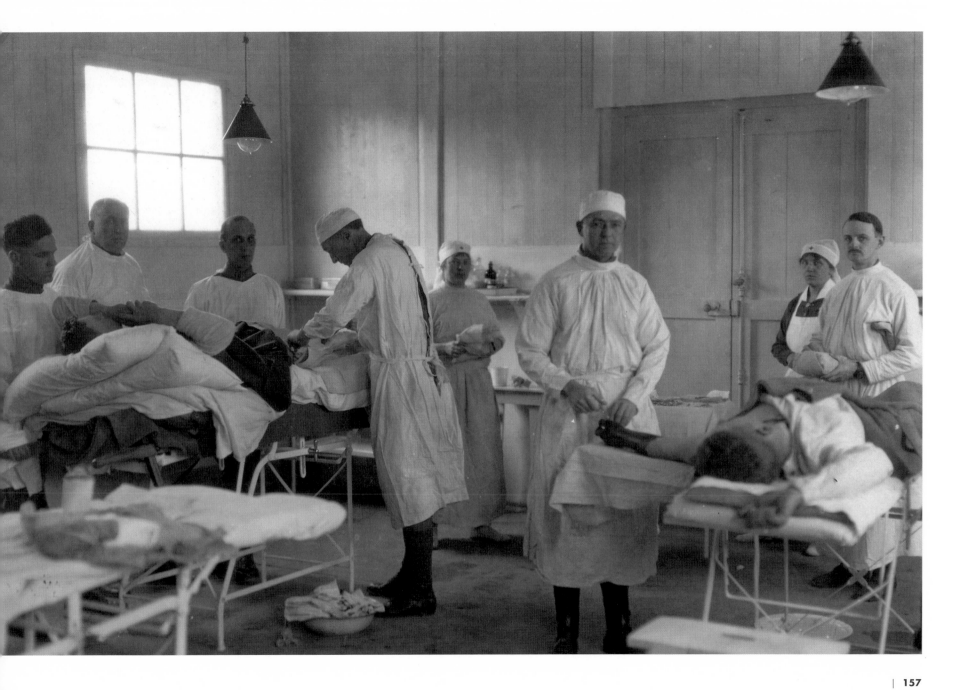

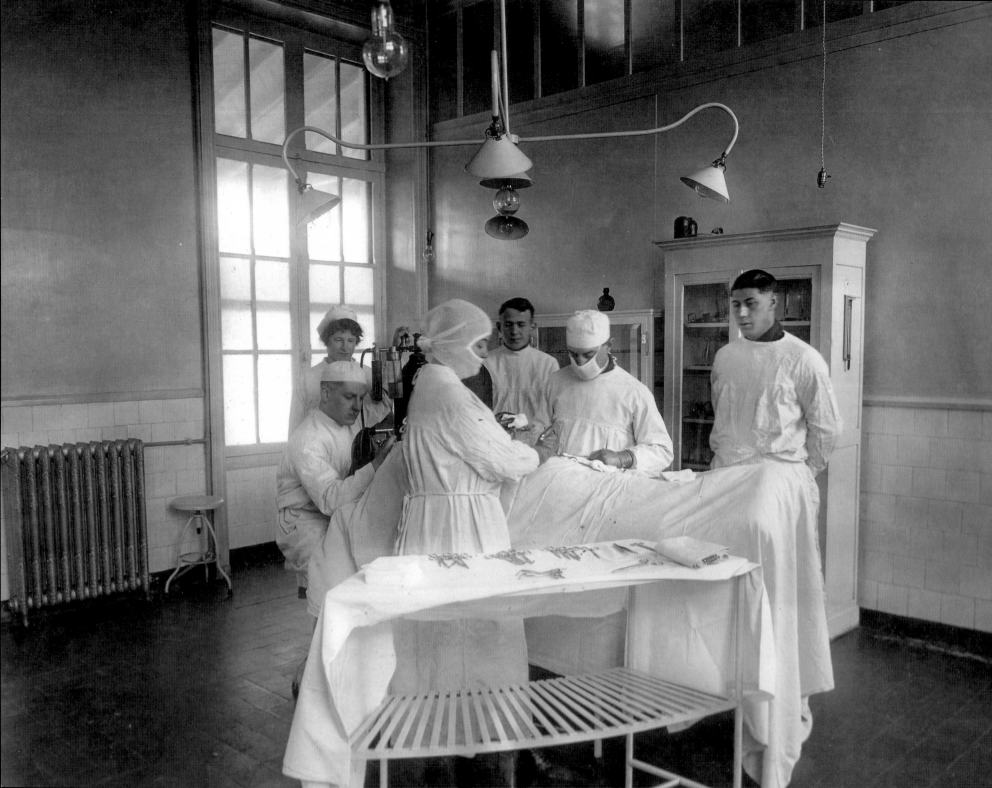

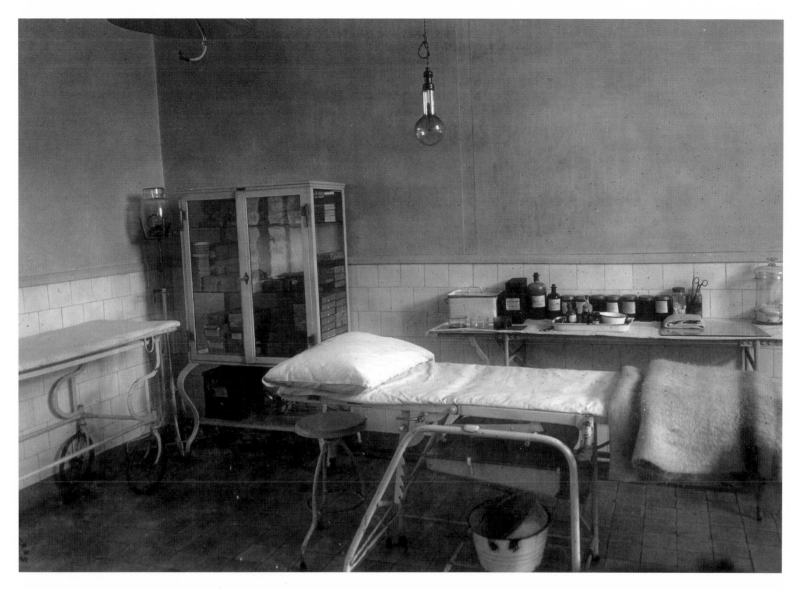

(Opposite) *Operating room with surgical staff, Base Hospital No. 101, St. Nazaire, France.*

(Above) *Dressing room at Base Hospital No. 101, St. Nazaire, France.*

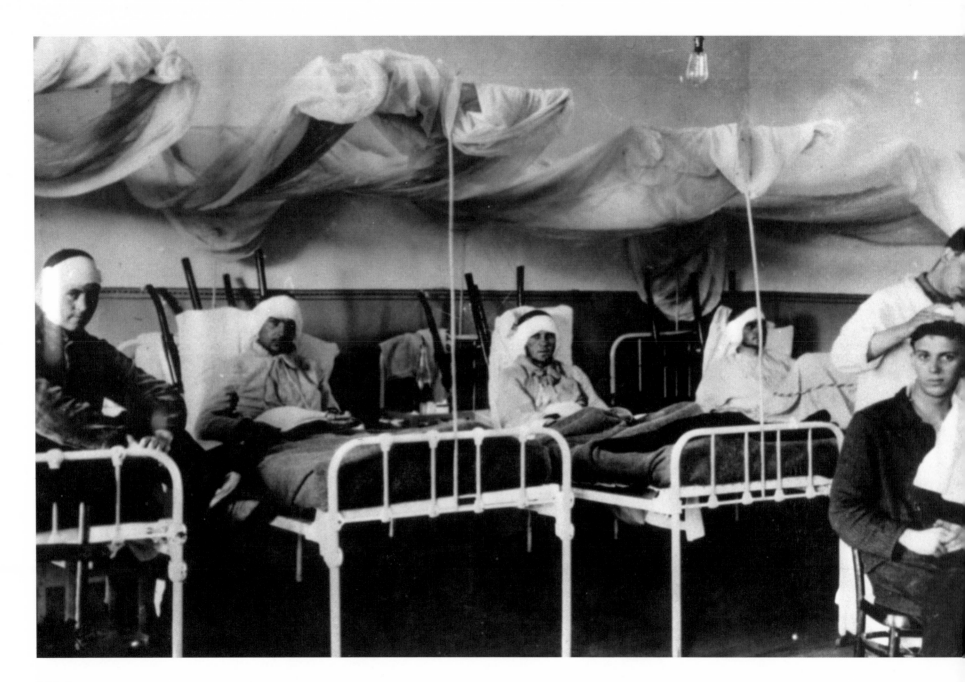

"In round numbers Base Hospital No. 101 has cared for about 20,000 patients. Statistics compiled from June 27 until the present time [1919] show that over 10,000 medical cases have been cared for and over 8,000 surgical cases. The latter include those orthopaedic cases, battle casualties, and minor cases evacuated from the advance hospital, and include the operative cases receiving attention in our surgery." (*Surgeon General Report, 1919, p. 2004*)

St. Nazaire was one of the main ports used by Allied forces. During the influenza epidemic, ocean transports arrived laden with great numbers of ill, many of whom had died at sea. Medical staff at hospitals in the St. Nazaire area were exhausted from overwork and nightly vigil as they struggled to cope with so many cases of severe pneumonia. The number of deaths was "quite appalling." (*Surgeon General Report, 1919, p. 2004*)

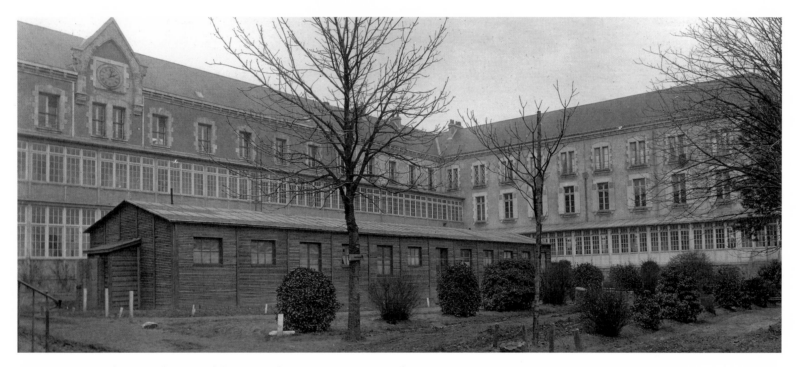

(Opposite) *Ward No. 4 ("A"), used for mastoid cases at Base Hospital No. 101, St. Nazaire, France. June 25, 1918.*

(Above) *Base Hospital No. 101, St. Nazaire, France.*

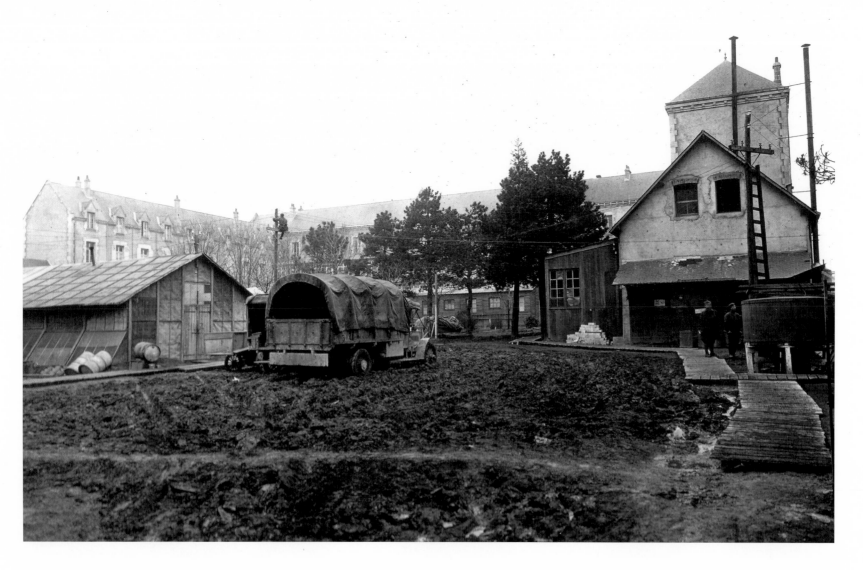

(Above) *Rear views of Base Hospital No. 101, St. Nazaire, France.*

(Opposite) *Front headquarters building, Base Hospital No.101.*

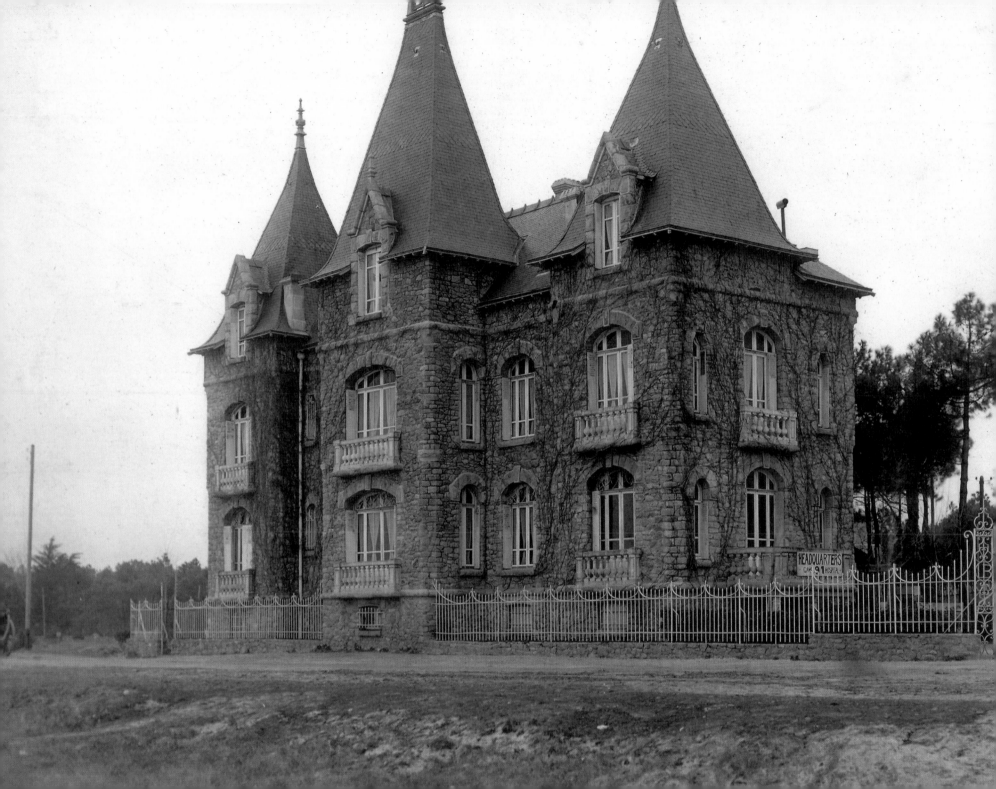

"The first train of wounded battle casualties arrived on June 11 [1918] from the Chateau-Thierry sector, and consisted of about 60 mildly gassed cases, 77 wounded stretcher cases, and the remainder of the 250 walking cases." By August, numbers rose to 412 wounded arriving by train from Chateau-Thierry. "By using seven Quartermaster Corps ambulances, three Ford ambulances, and a number of 3-ton trucks (patients in double tier), all were transported a distance of a mile and in the hospital within two and one-half hours." *(Surgeon General Report, 1919, p. 2005)*

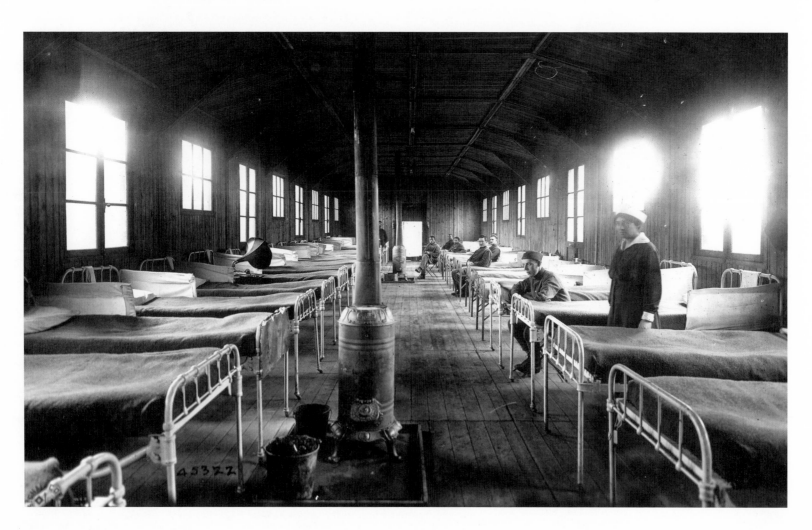

(Opposite) *Ward 11 (medical), Base Hospital No. 101, St. Nazaire, France.*

(Below) *Nurses of Base Hospital No. 101.*

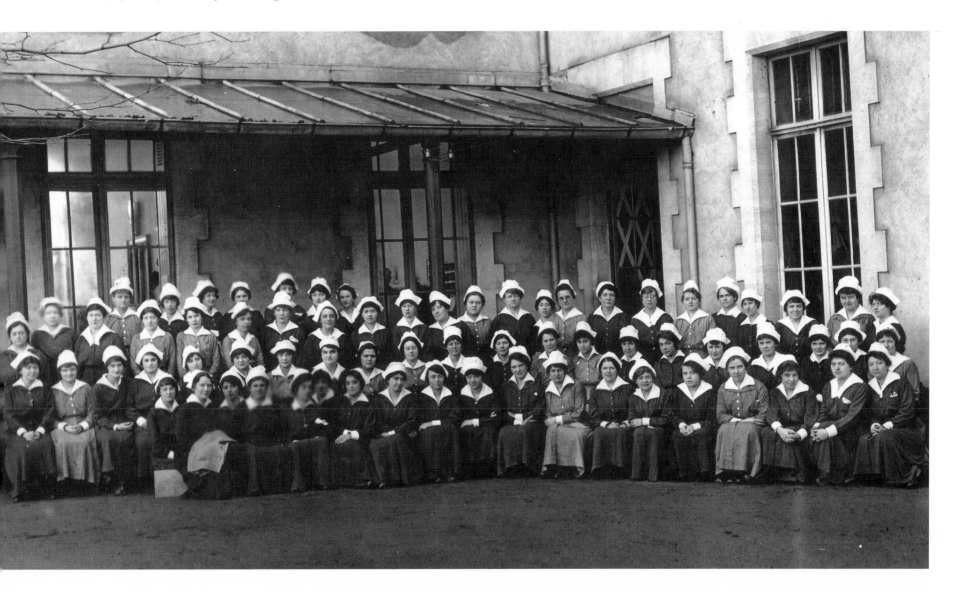

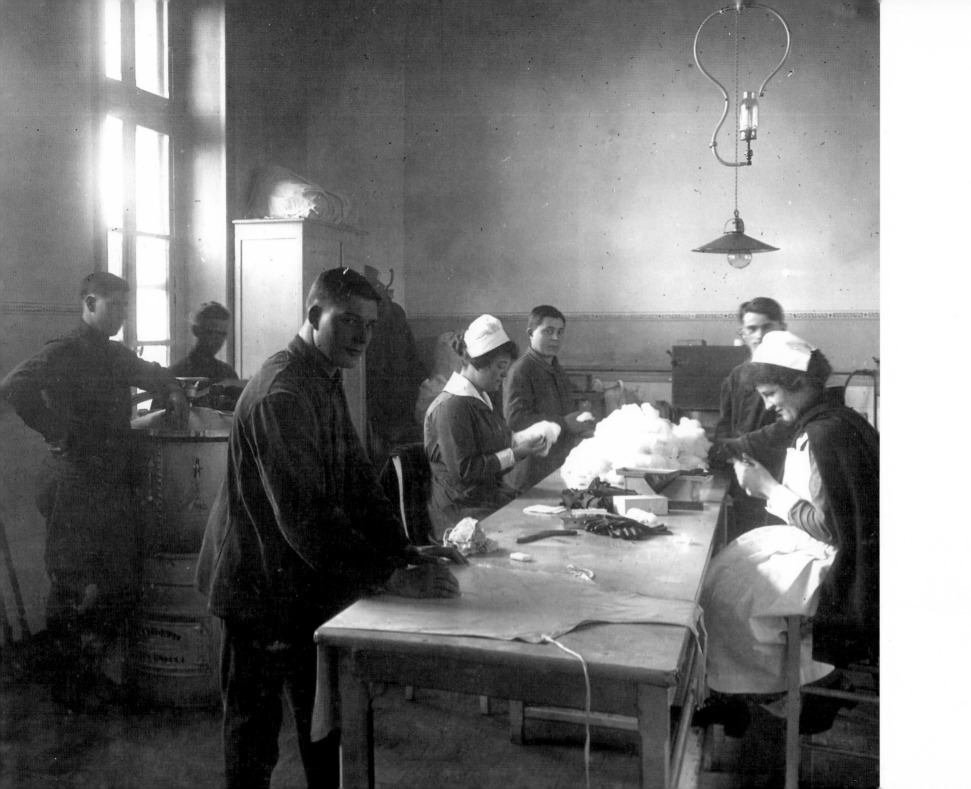

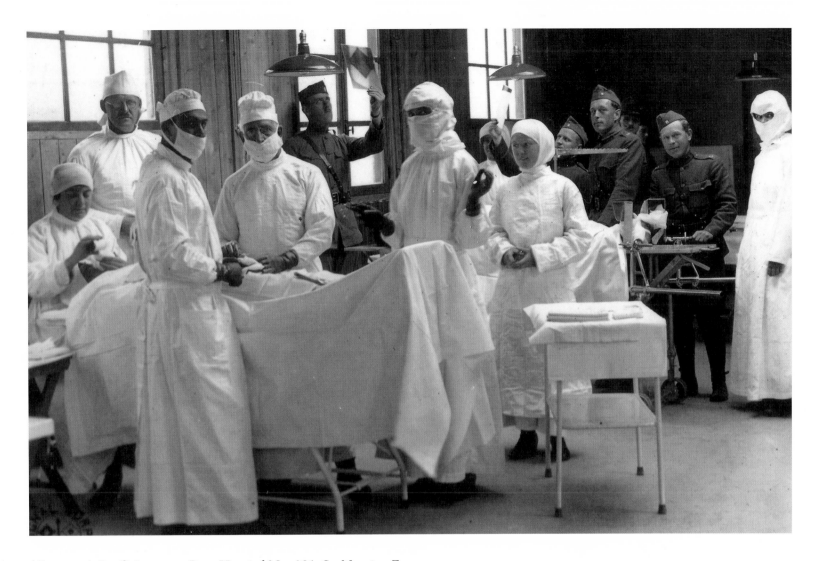

(Opposite) *Sterilizing room, Base Hospital No. 101, St. Nazaire, France.*

(Above) *View of the "new" operating room at Hospital Unit No. 116, which opened just days before this photograph was taken on June 15, 1918. Lieutenant Colonel Wolkes and Major Hold in charge. Aulnois-sous-Vertuzey (near Commercy, Meuse, France).*

Central Medical Department Laboratory

"This laboratory was established at Dijon, January 1, 1918, by officers from Army Laboratory No. 1, Neufchateau. The building for the purpose was donated by the University of Dijon at a nominal rent of 1 franc per year. At the time, with the exception of two laboratories in use by the university, the interior of the building was unfinished. Authorization was obtained and early in February the entire interior was reconstructed into a modern laboratory building and completely equipped with material brought from the States.

In March, 1918, the staff consisted of 16 officers, 35 enlisted men, and 12 civilian employees. The buildings then consisted of the large laboratory building, four barracks donated by the Red Cross which housed the office of the director of laboratories, a large lab for instruction of student officers, five well-equipped research labs, an operating room for experimental surgical research on animals, a complete X-ray installation and photographic darkroom, space for the art museum section, and a mess and quarters for the enlisted personnel." Other buildings were later added. (*Surgeon General Report, 1919, p. 1317*)

☙❦❧

"The supply division of this laboratory was charged with assembling, equipping, and issuing transportable lab equipment to mobile units; replenishing expendable items and replacing those that had become unserviceable; issuing to mobile units and camp hospitals various culture media and reagents required for bacteriologic work in the field; and issuing to all Medical Department units in the geographic region served by the Central Medical Department laboratory the various biological products used in the diagnosis prevention and treatment of infectious diseases.

During the period of active participation of our troops at the front, the greater portion of these supplies was delivered by courier service, necessitating the constant operation of numerous camionettes, trucks, and motor cycles." (*The Medical Dept in the World War, p. 1319*)

(Opposite) *Central Medical Laboratory set up in Dijon, France. September 1918.*

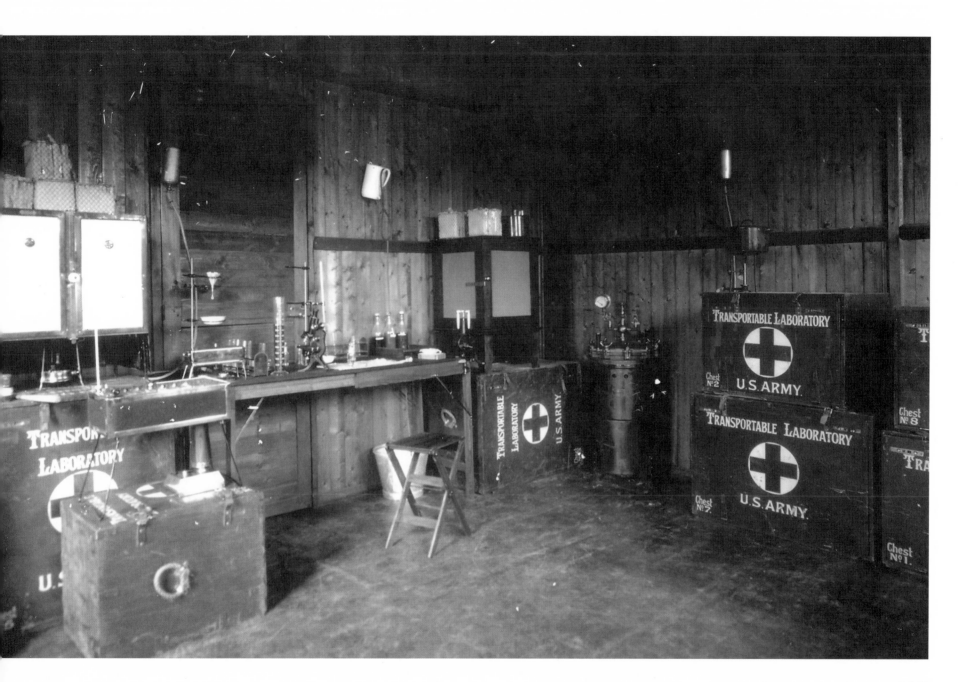

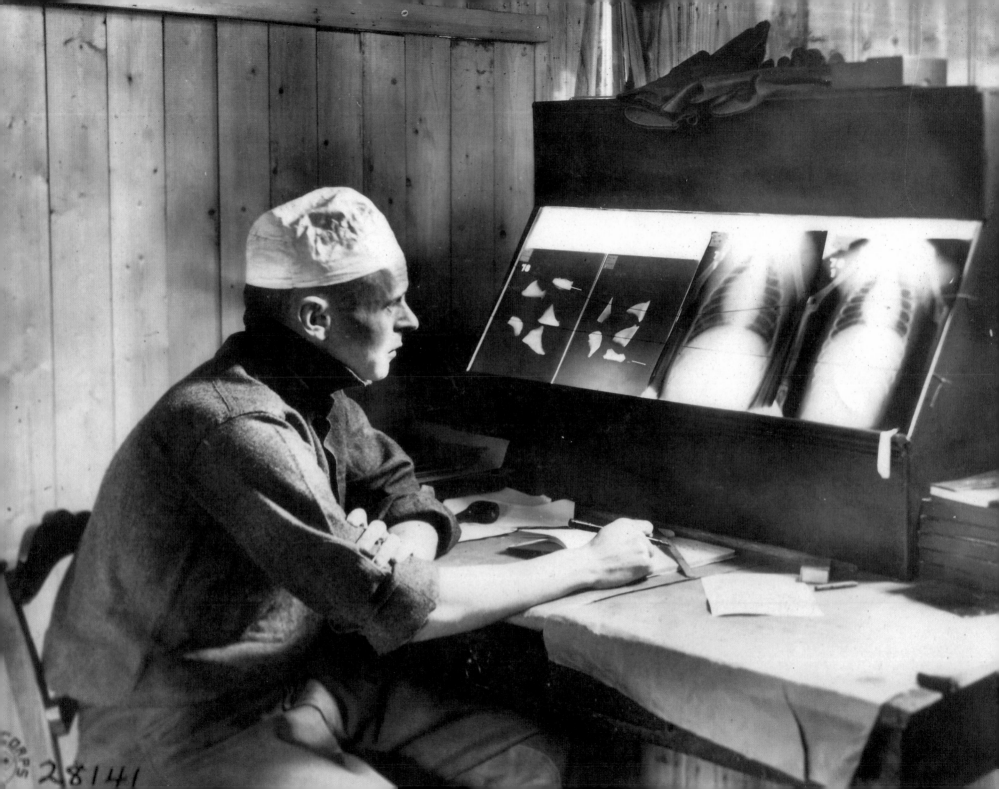

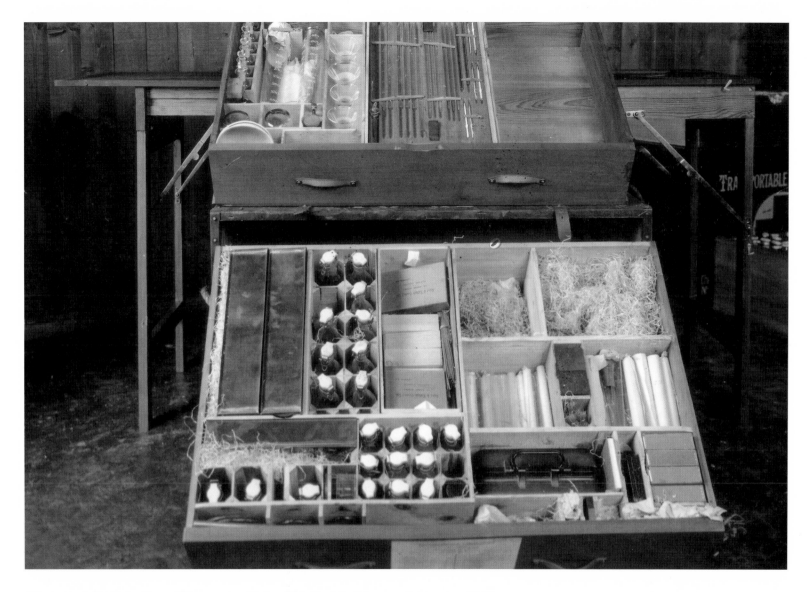

(Opposite) *Captain Gray, X-ray room, Central Medical Laboratory, September 1918.*

(Above) *Chest number one ready for transport, Central Medical Department Laboratory.*

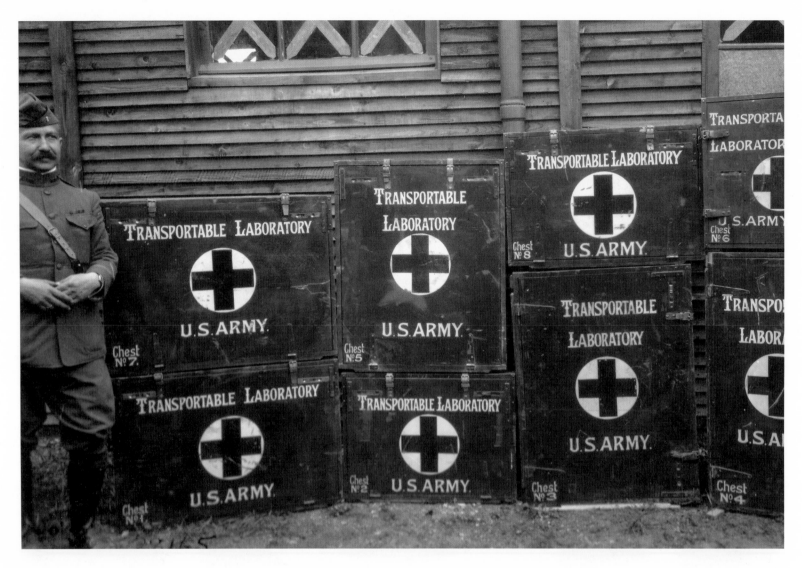

(Above) *Lieutenant Bitterman and eight laboratory chests, Central Medical Department Laboratory.*

(Opposite) *Laboratory store room, Dijon, France*

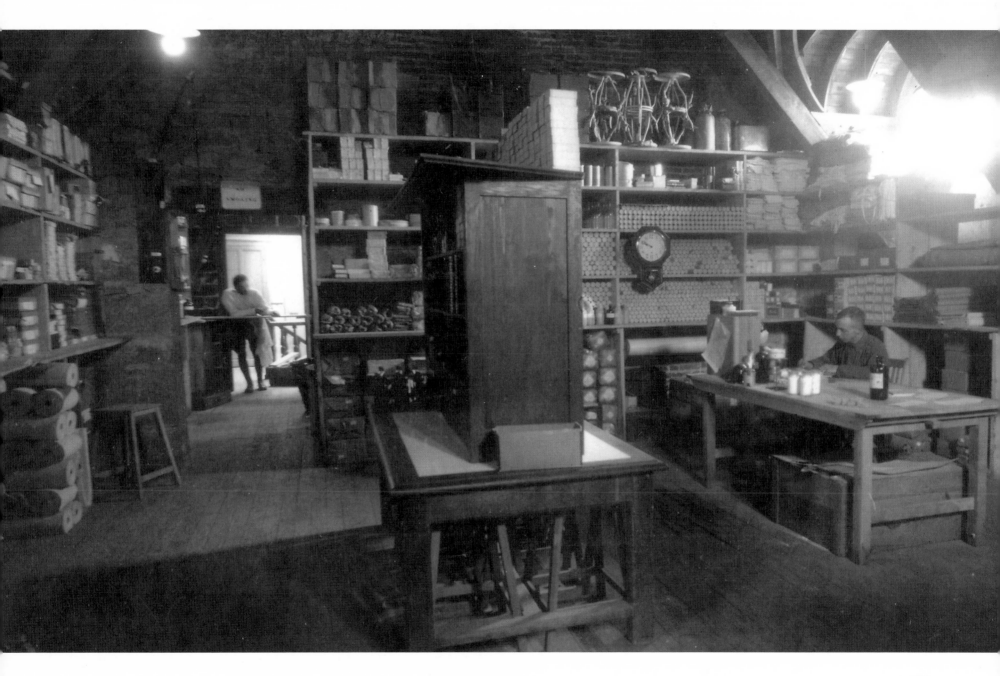

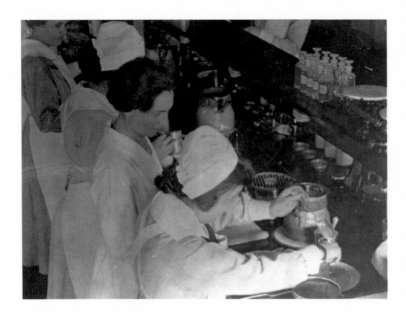

(Above) *Nurses performing laboratory work somewhere in France.*

(Right) *Interior of field laboratory car, Central Medical Laboratory, Dijon, France. September 1918.*

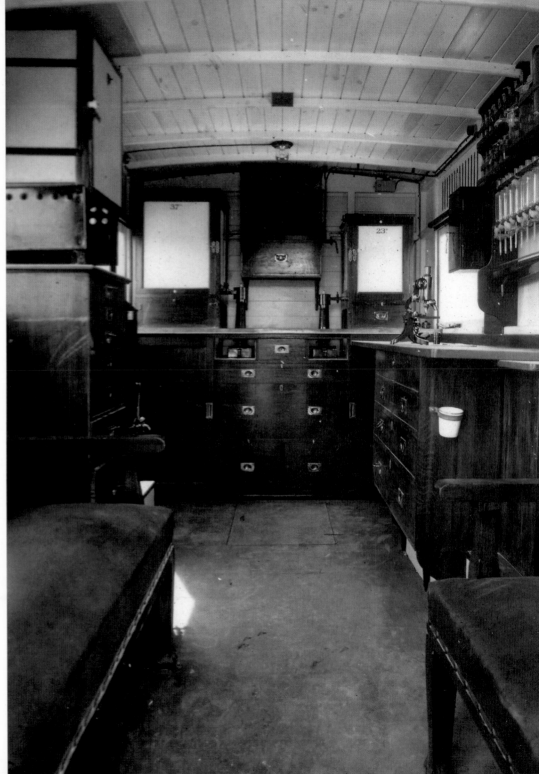

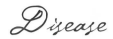

Disease

In the United States

"THE HEALTH OF TROOPS WAS EXCELLENT up to the latter part of September, when the epidemic of influenza-pneumonia appeared in our eastern camps. At the beginning of July 1918, the annual death rate for disease was 3.1 per 1,000. During the latter part of September, with the appearance of the influenza/pneumonia epidemic, mortality rates soared. All previous records for mortality from disease among the troops in camps were shattered. During the peak period of the epidemic, reached in mid-October, the rate was 206.4 deaths per 1,000.

The influenza-pneumonia epidemic was a world-wide calamity. The number of deaths caused by the disease throughout the world in 1918 is variously estimated. It is certain that deaths were numbered in the millions, one estimate stating that 6,000,000 fatalities occurred within the period of the last six months of 1918." *(Surgeon General Report, 1919, p. 1033)*

Overseas

"Early in September cases of influenza and pneumonia began to arrive on the transports. During this period very few ships arrived without cases of either of these diseases. The total number of cases of influenza arriving during the months of September and October were [*sic*] 4,187, and of pneumonia 913. Too much stress can not be laid on the exactness of these figures; for many of the cases called influenza later proved to be pneumonia; nor do they give an adequate idea of the number of cases actually occurring on the ships, for many cases of influenza went to duty before they reached port. Nor do these figures include those that died en route, of which there were no less than 479, nor those that, having been infected on board, developed the disease in Pontanezen rest camp and either recovered or died. The total number of deaths occurring after landing here, from pneumonia alone, has been about 1,217." *(Surgeon General Report, 1919, p. 2050)*

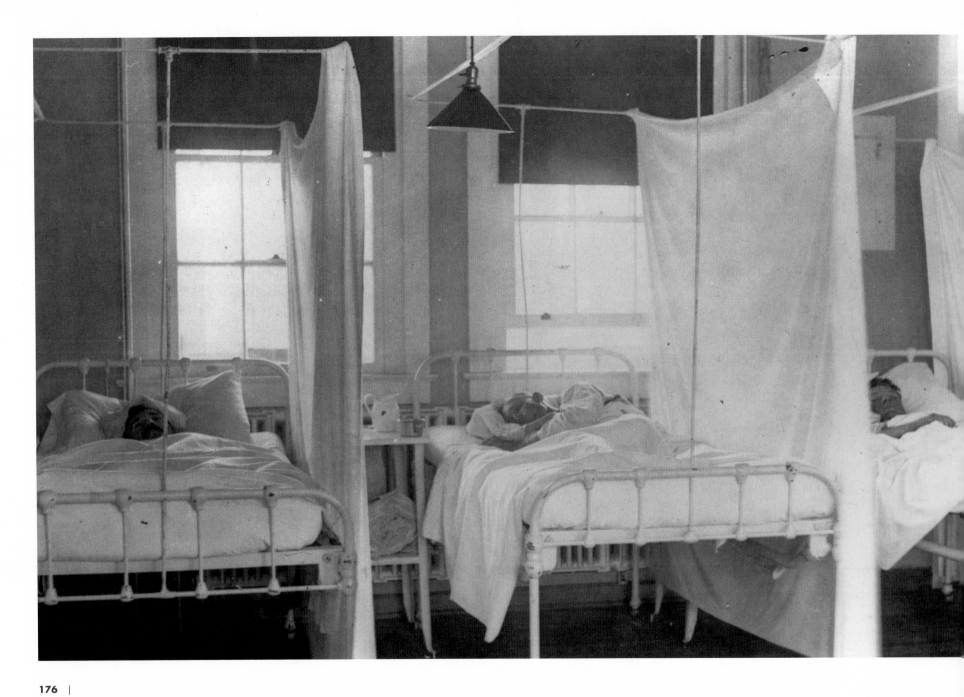

"October 9th [1918]: Haven't written in this diary from Sept 25. Had an epidemic called Spanish grip. It has been awful. The hospital was increased to several thousand more beds. Barracks used also. So that they accommodated over 7,000 patients. In the beginning ten nurses were called to NY. . . . The death rate has been awful. Up to this date their [*sic*] must have been over 700 deaths. Some awful and depressing. Was all in myself but kept up. On duty until 12 every night. Six boys in the wd [ward] to help out and two night nurses. Supplies ran low. People of Rockford [Illinois] helped in every way. The boys slept in tents with a stove & electric lights. Some of the old boys that I know passed away." (*Diary of Jocobina R. Riecke, R.N., ANC, Camp Grant, Illinois*)

The influenza epidemic spread throughout the training camps in the United States, demanding new levels of patient care. The Red Cross worked to recruit enough emergency detachments to fill the camps' requirements. Nursing personnel of the base hospital units waiting for deployment overseas were reassigned to the camps. This gave them preliminary training in a military hospital and also gave hospitals an adequate nursing staff.

In the United States, 127 Army nurses died as a result of influenza. (*Sarnecky, p. 121*)

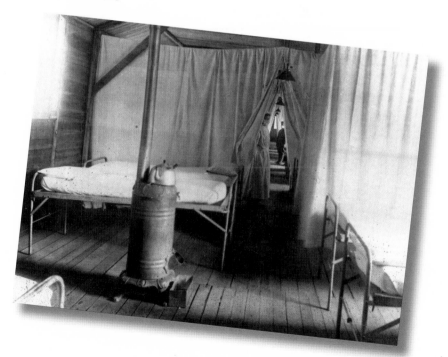

(Opposite) *Pneumonia Ward at Walter Reed Army Hospital, circa 1919.*

(Right) *Infectious Disease Ward, Base Hospital No. 59, Rimacourt, France.*

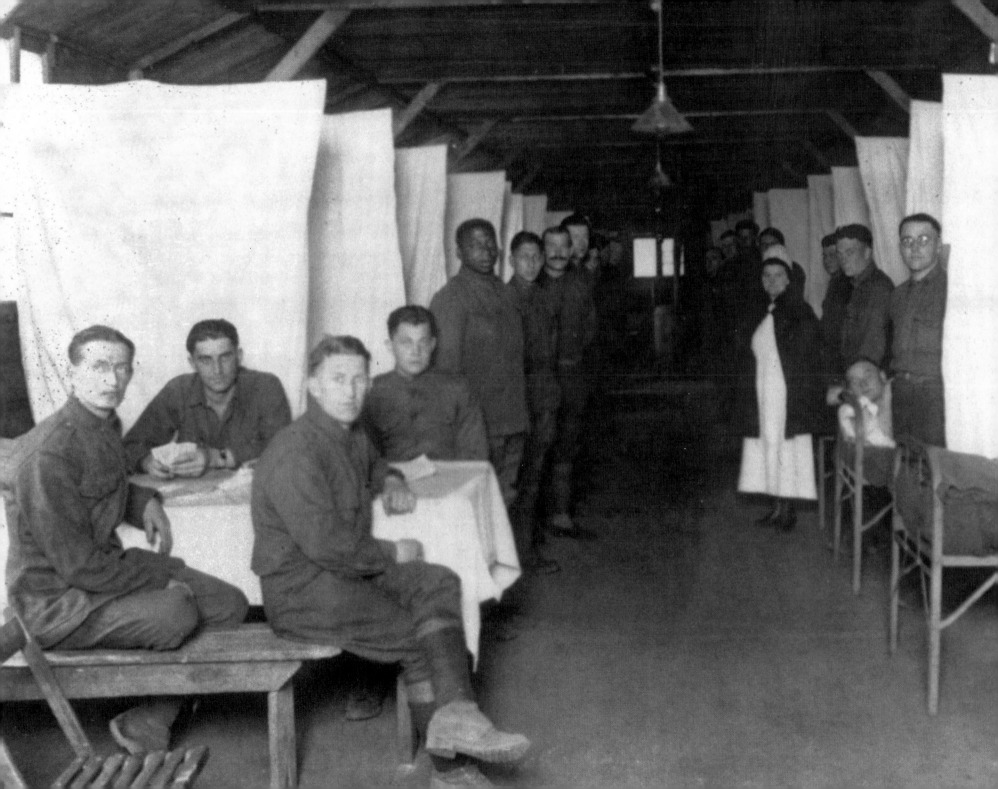

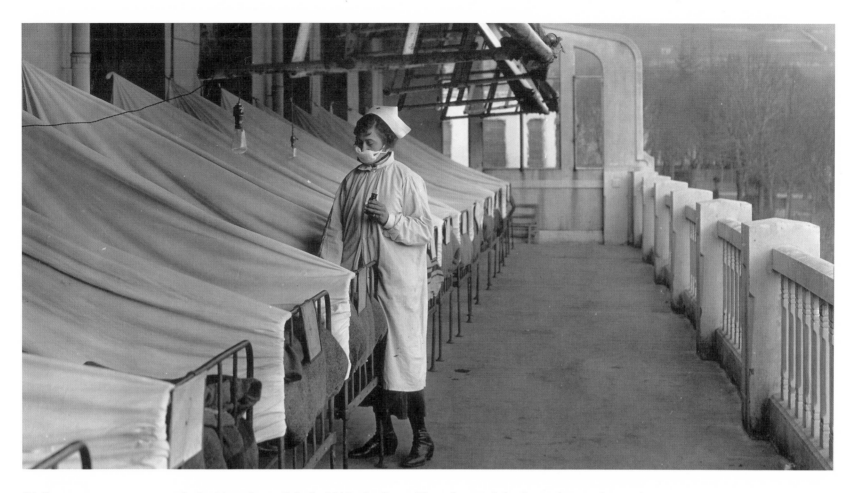

"Following negotiations with the French, on July 8, 1918, the Leon Blanc hospital, built on the outskirts of Aix-les-Bains in 1912, was officially transferred to the American Expeditionary Forces as Camp Hospital No. 45. The three large porches accommodated the pneumonias and were doubtless responsible to a large degree for the low death rate here, which averaged about 17.5 per cent. It was noticed that most of the fatal cases were of a peculiarly rapid and virulent mixed infection, resulting in a very massive form of pneumonia." (*Surgeon General Report, 1919, p. 2117*)

(Opposite) *Medical Contagious Ward, Base Hospital No. 64, Rimacourt, France, 1919.*

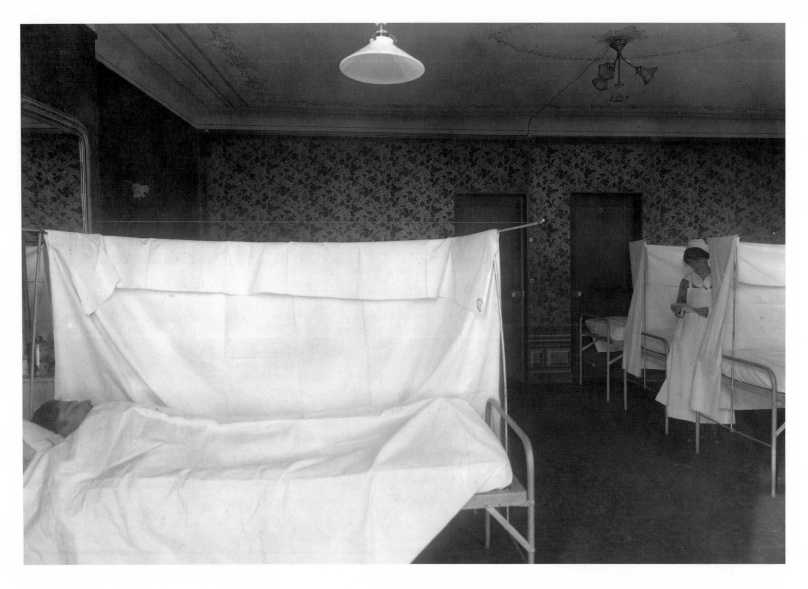

(Above) *Influenza patient in the Observation Ward, Hotel Costebelle, Base Hospital No. 99, Hyeres, France.*

(Opposite) *Tuberculosis Ward at Hotel Metropole, Base Hospital No. 93.*

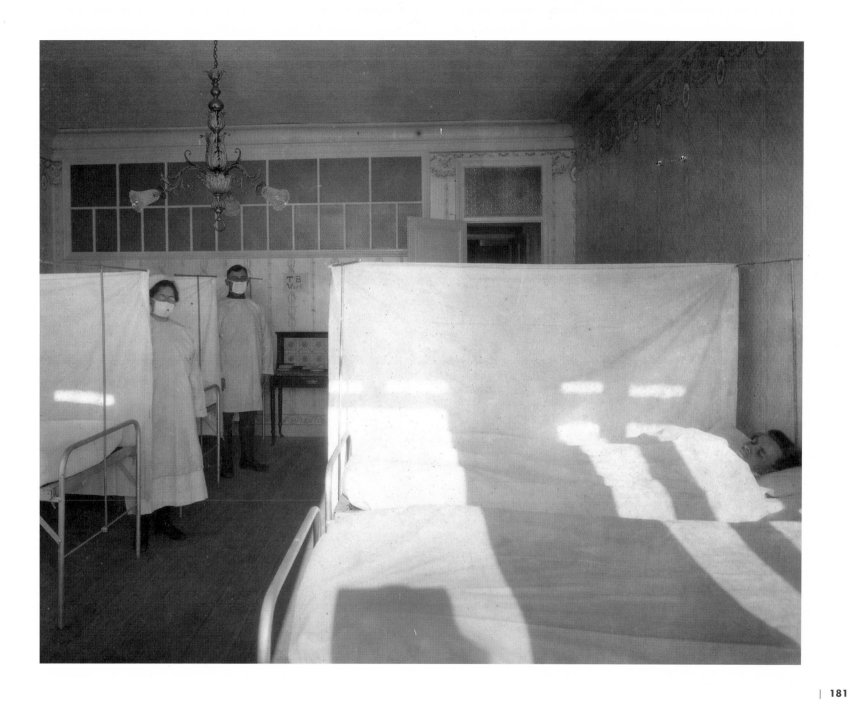

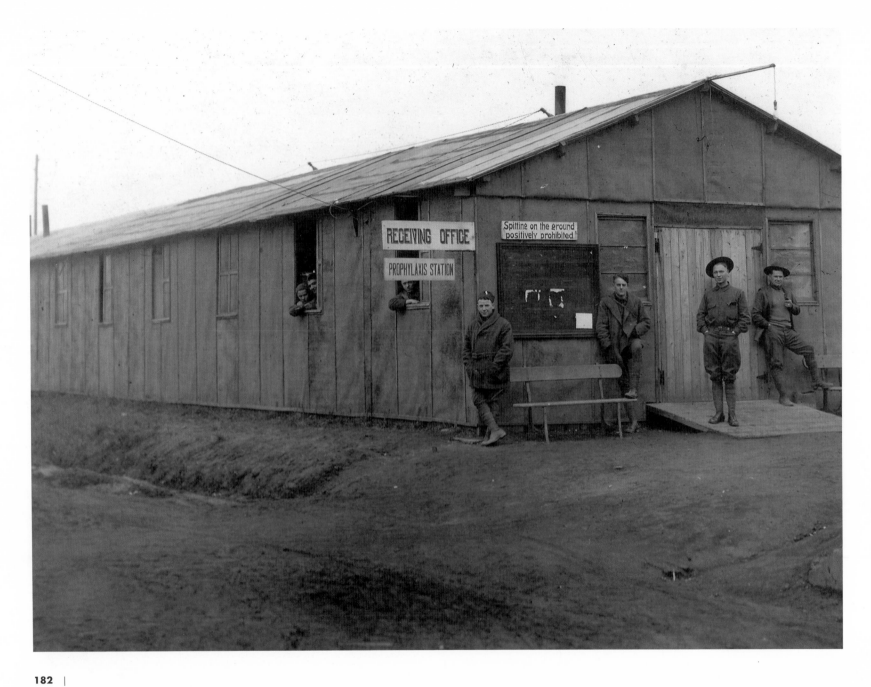

Venereal Diseases

"Venereal diseases have been subject to control by policies, medical, educational, and disciplinary, so different from those applied in any Army heretofore. . . . It is not too much to say that the official attitude of the Government as expressed in orders from the War Department and from the commander in chief supported by a logical medical service for the prevention and treatment of venereal diseases, have resulted in a smaller loss of man power to the Army, a lower incidence rate of the diseases, and a small number of permanently disabled and invalided men from these diseases than has been recorded in any other army up to the present time. . . .

These diseases, when treated according to the information available through medical science, can be controlled, and to a greater degree than ever before have been controlled, by applying the principles of preventive medicine, namely, diminution of contact with human sources of infection, prophylactic treatment promptly after exposure, and segregation with intensive treatment for those in the communicable stages of the diseases."
(Report of the Surgeon General, 1919, p. 1312)

*(Opposite)Exterior receiving office, which also served as the "prophylaxis station,"
Base Hospital No. 101, St. Nazaire, France.*

Subcutaneous emphysema occurs when air gets into tissues under the skin covering the chest wall or neck. This can happen due to stabbing, gunshot wounds, other penetrations, or blunt trauma. Air can also be found between skin layers on the arms and legs during certain infections, including gas gangrene. When a healthcare provider touches the skin, it produces an unusual crackling sensation as the gas is pushed through the tissue.

(Left and Opposite) *Mendell's application was used in conjunction with open air treatment to treat wounds for subcutaneous emphysema. Date and place unknown.*

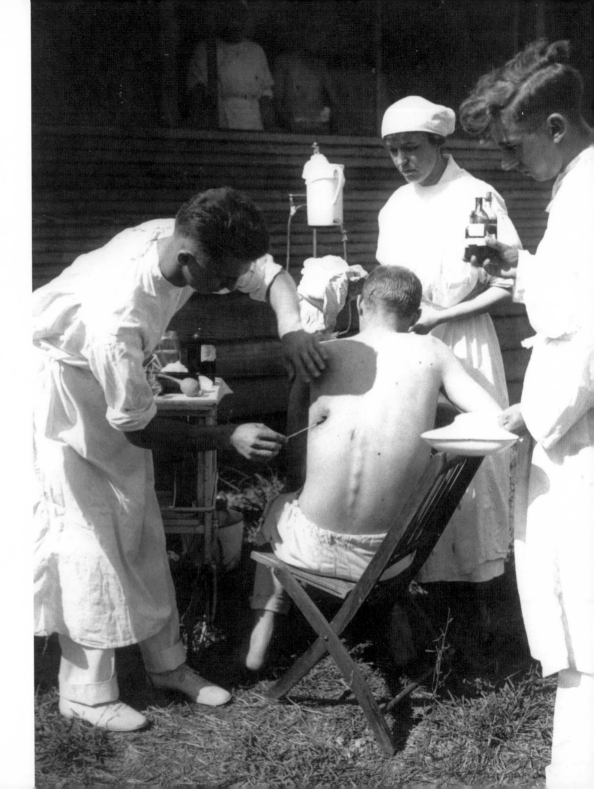

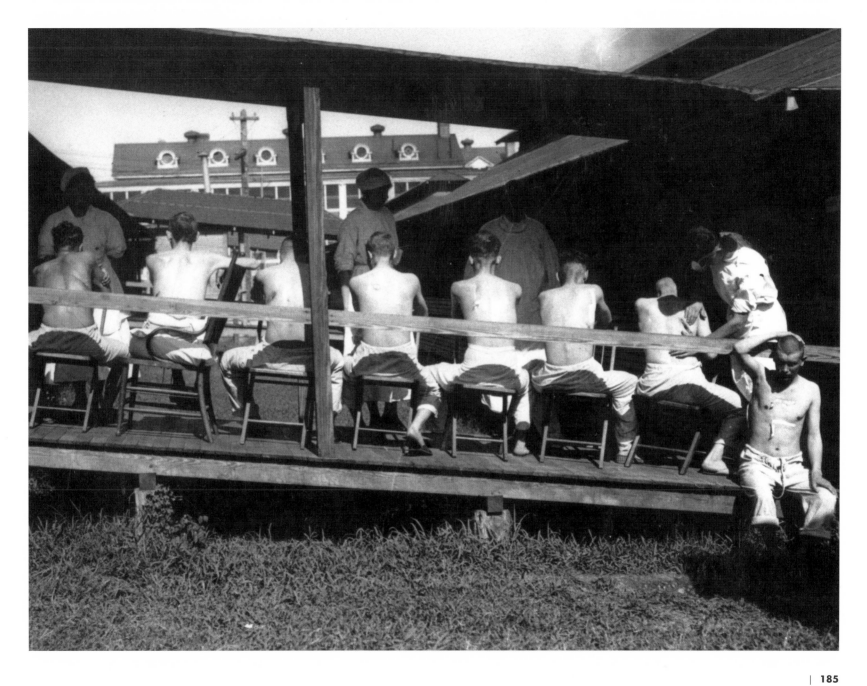

Death

THE AMERICAN GRAVES REGISTRATION SERVICE reported approximately 81,067 overseas war deaths by the armistice. However, casualty figures vary considerably, making it difficult to precisely determine actual combat fatalities. The figure often quoted, approximately 50,510, reflects combat fatalities and does not include influenza or accident victims. A total of 30,902 casualties were buried in European cemeteries, and 46,304 bodies were returned to the United States.

"Members of the Army Nurse Corps who died during their Army service were buried with military honors. In November, 1918, a plot in Arlington National Cemetery was assigned for the burial of Army nurses and since that time nurses have been buried there if their families so desired." *(The Medical Dept in the World War, Vol. XIII p. 311)*

"On the whole the health of nurses in the American Expeditionary Forces was very good. The influenza epidemic of 1918 affected members of the Nurse corps as it did the men of the Army. Only two nurses were wounded at all seriously, and none were killed by the enemy. By the time the first nurses in France had been there a year only six deaths had occurred among them, and at this time there were 2,500 nurses in the AEF. Up through August, 1918, there were 15 deaths, but in September there were 8 more, October, 41, and in November, 12. One was killed in an airplane accident, another was run over by a train, another was thrown from a horse, and a number were killed in automobile accidents." *(The Medical Dept in the World War, Vol. XIII, p. 350)*

"In the case of death among the nurses, upon the chief nurse fell the duty of writing to the parents and describing the details as best she might, of readjusting the duties among already overworked women, of assisting at funeral ceremonies, of keeping up morale, and also of arranging for the nursing of other sick members. It takes but little imagination to picture the frame of mind of a chief nurse who had gone through this process twelve times in one month, as once happened during the period of the influenza epidemic. The cumulative effect of so many funerals would have had serious consequences under normal conditions, and 3,000 miles from home, in a foreign land without the usual means of diversion, it took strong character to withstand the pressure." *(The Medical Dept in the World War, Vol. XIII, p. 345)*

(Opposite) *Graveside service in 1917 showing women of the Army Nurse Corps wearing the uniform first authorized to nurses going overseas.*

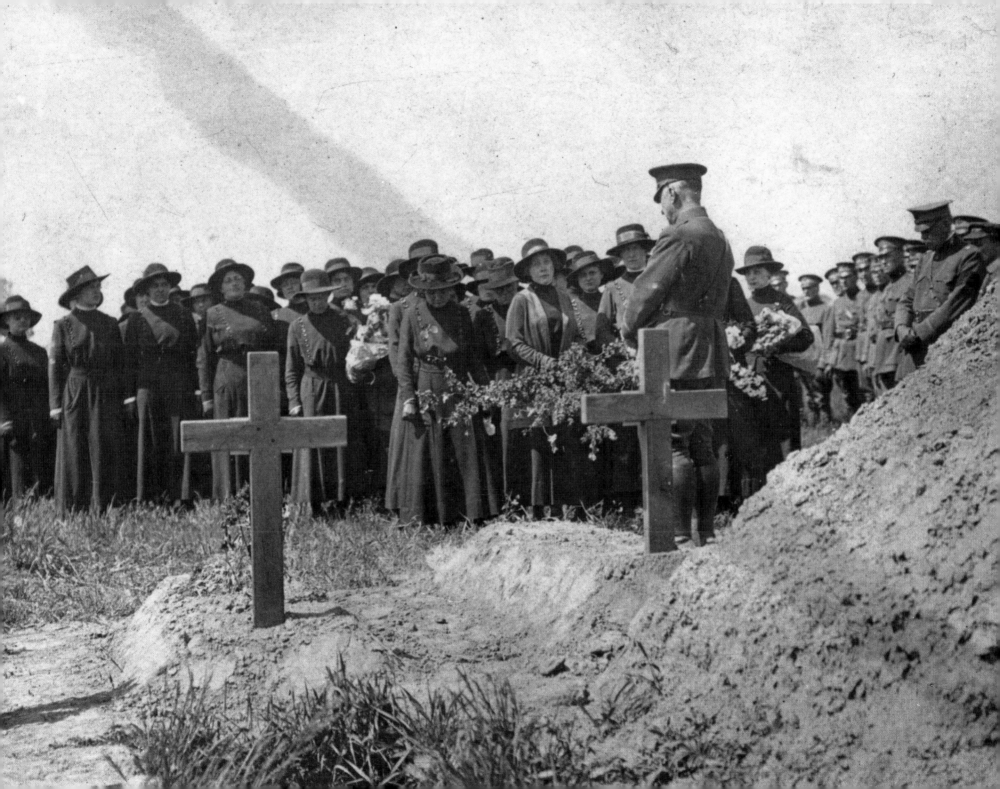

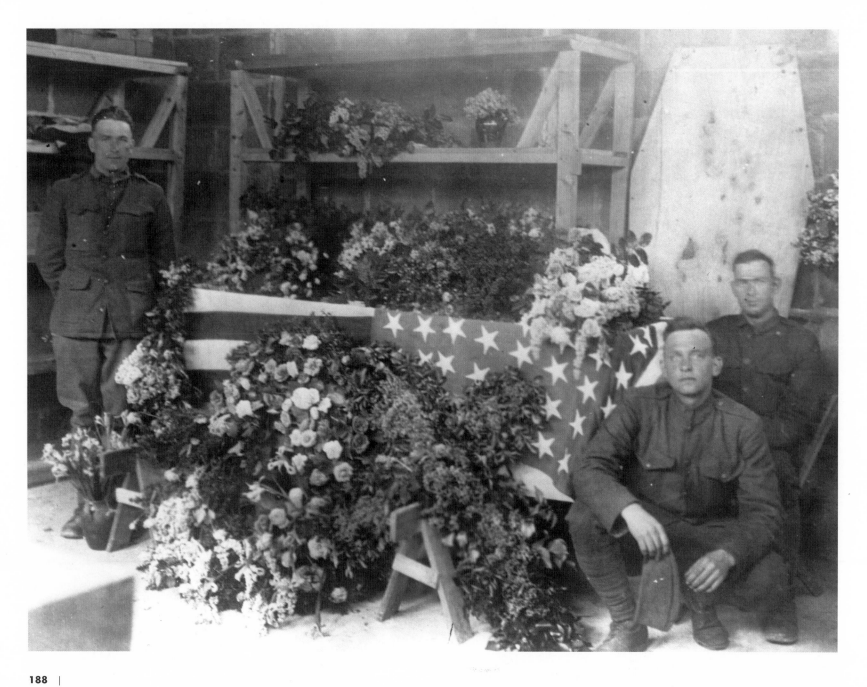

Jane Delano sailed to France at the end of December 1918 on official Red Cross business. In February 1919, she and Julia Stimson traveled throughout the country speaking to nurses until she fell ill with a middle ear infection at Savenay. The infection progressed into mastoiditis and later required surgery. By March she developed a brain abscess, which required further surgery from which Delano never regained consciousness. She died on April 15, 1919, and was buried in Savenay. In 1920 Delano's body was exhumed, returned to the United States, and reinterred in the nurses' plot at Arlington National Cemetery in Virginia. *(Sarnecky, p. 133)*

The U.S. government awarded Delano the Distinguished Service Medal posthumously.

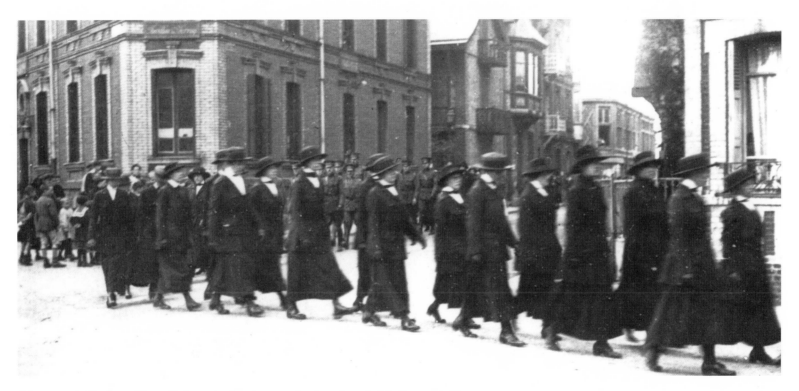

(Opposite) *Casket of Jane Delano in the morgue of a base hospital in Savenay, France.*

(Above) *Funeral procession for an Army nurse who died in France, date and location unknown.*

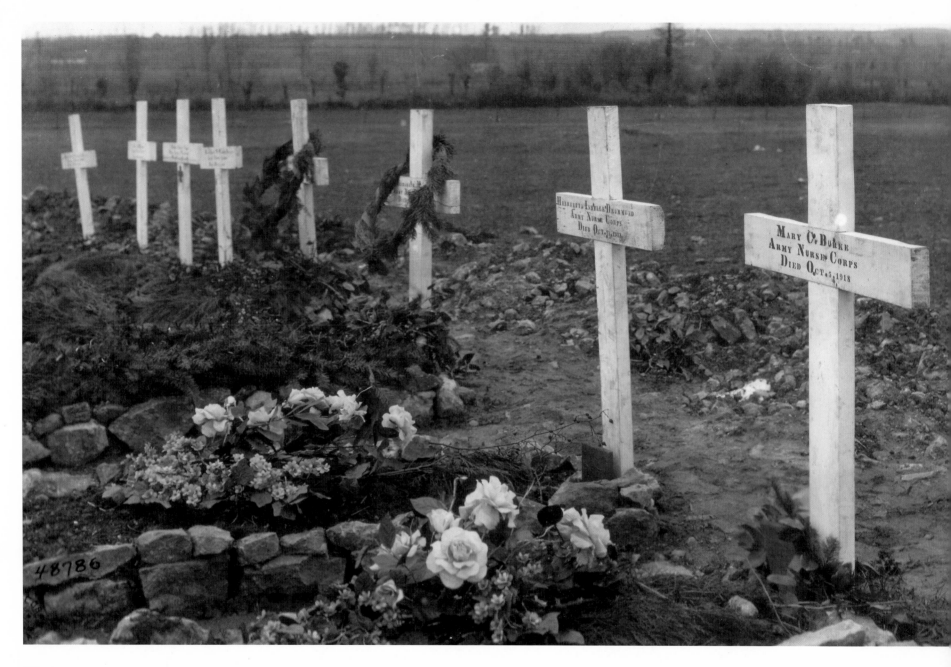

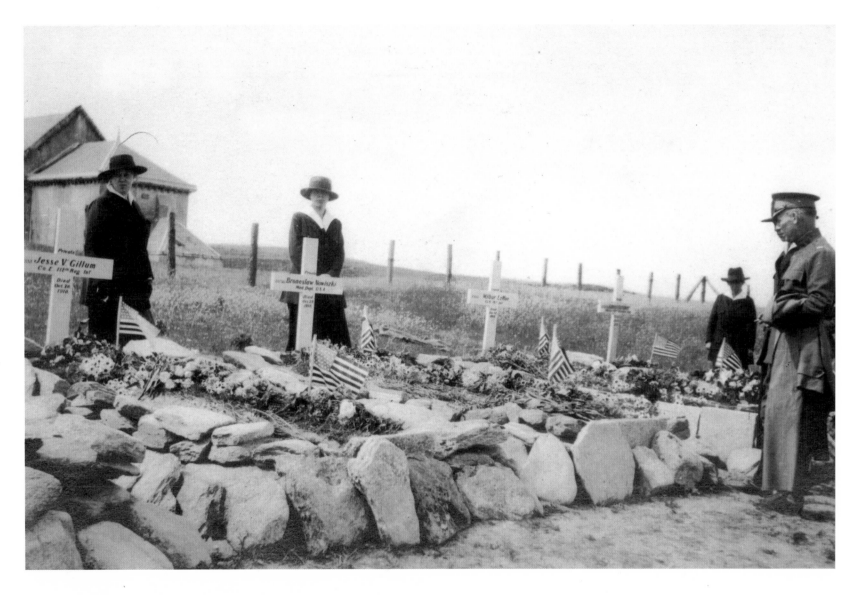

(Opposite) *Nurses' graves at a hospital cemetery at Mars-sur-Allier, Nievre, France. January 1919.*

(Above) *View of the American Expeditionary Forces Cemetery at Quiberon, situated on a peninsula on the French coast in Brittany.*

Army nurse Helen Fairchild, from Pennsylvania, volunteered to go overseas with 63 other nurses from Pennsylvania Hospital just one month after the United States declared war in April 1917. She was 32 years old when she served with Base Hospital No. 10, stationed at Le Treport, France.

Fairchild had had a history of abdominal pain before she left for France, and during November 1917 she suffered from a recurrence. By Christmas she was vomiting after every meal, and in January X-rays and exploratory surgery revealed a massive gastric ulcer, caused or worsened by exposure to mustard gas used by the enemy. She underwent a gastro-enterostomy on January 13, 1918, and initially did well but became jaundiced on the third day postoperative and deteriorated rapidly. She died in a coma on January 18, 1918.

Fairchild's cause of death was initially attributed to acute atrophy of the liver, but a post-mortem examination showed the final cause of death to be hepatic complications of the chloroform used for her general anaesthetic.

Fairchild received a full military funeral attended by an entire garrison of English, Canadian, French, and American officers, nurses, and troops. She was buried first in Mont Huron Cemetery, Le Treport, and later reburied in the American Cemetery at Bony (Somme), France. (Rote, Nurse Helen Fairchild, WW1 1917-1918)

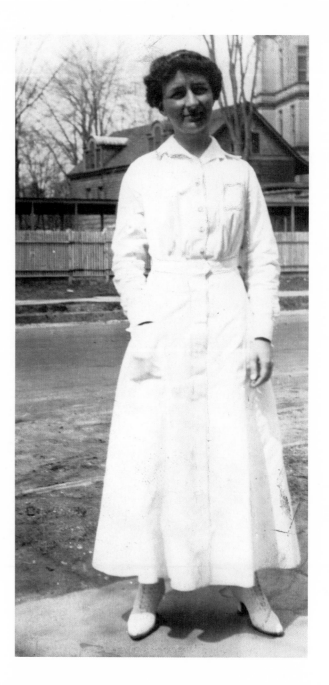

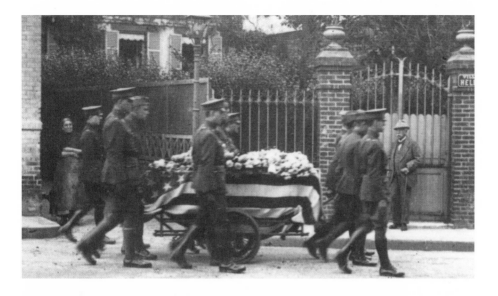

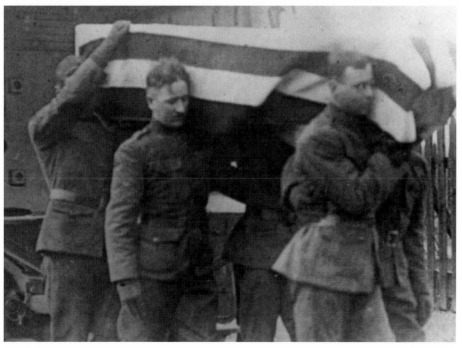

"The bodies were taken to the military cemetery in ambulances driven by women from the motor convoy. Sometimes, always in the case of American burials, the chaplain headed the procession from the mortuary, and sometimes he met the funeral cortege at the entrance of the cemetery. The burial party consisted of the chaplain, one or more officers and an escort of men under a non-commissioned officer. The men carried the coffins from the cemetery gate to the grave on their shoulders and then stood at attention during the service until taps or the last-post had been sounded. . . . One of the most impressive funerals in our experience was that of nurse Helen Fairchild who was buried on January 19, 1918. Every officer, nurse, motor-driver and enlisted man that could be spared from duty attended the service. Every hospital in the group was largely represented." *(Pennsylvania Hospital Unit in the Great War, 1921)*

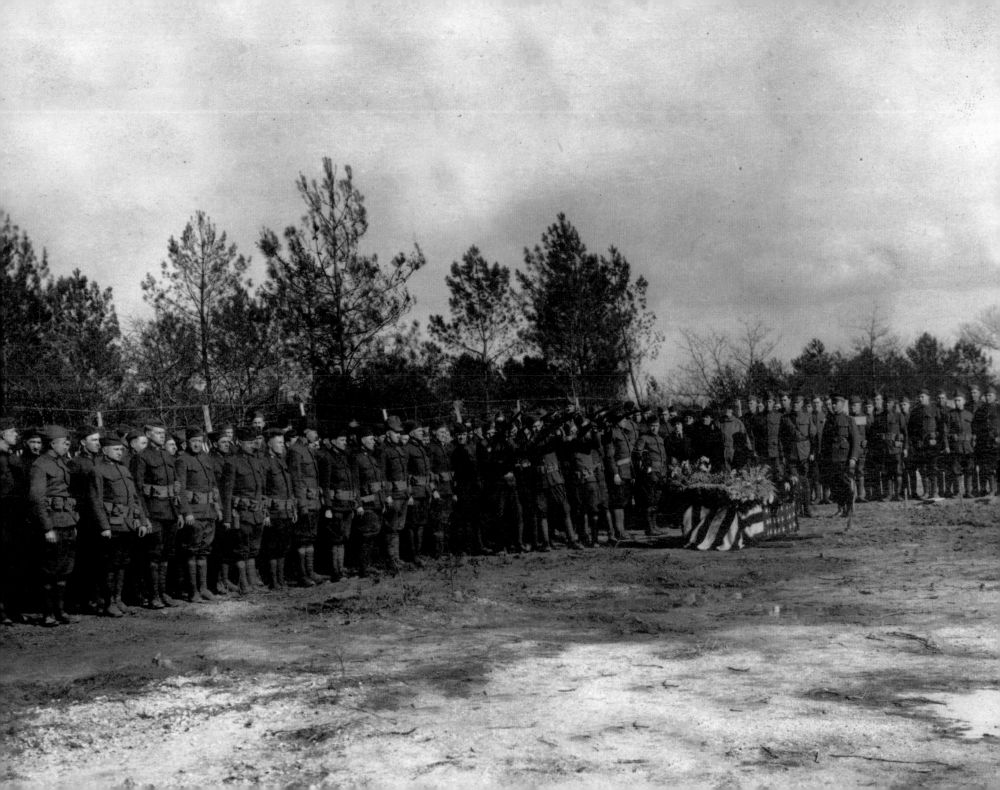

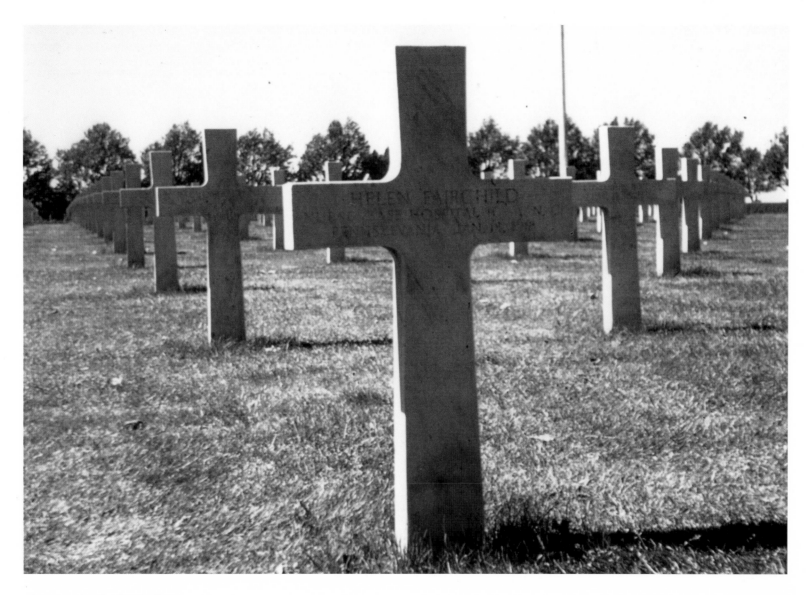

(Opposite) *The final salute.*

(Above) *The American Cemetery at Bony, France.*

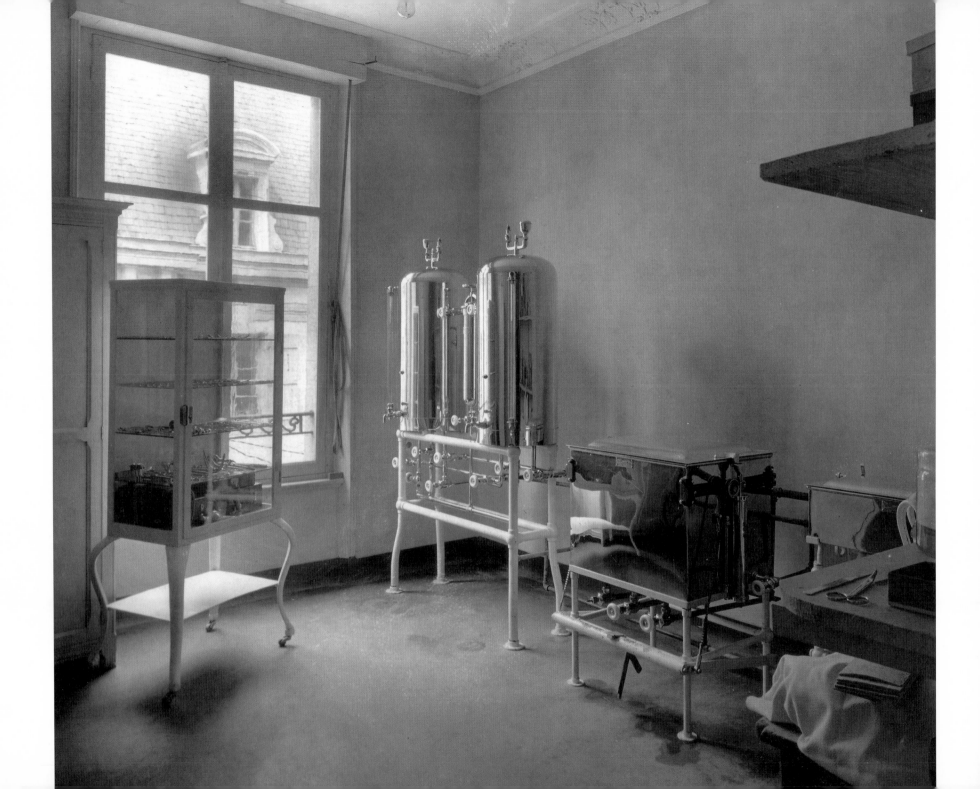

Hospital Centers

SOON AFTER THE ARRIVAL OF AMERICAN TROOPS IN FRANCE, the Medical Department recognized the need for economizing on the transportation of medical supplies and the movement of sick and wounded from the battlefront, as well as the benefits of combining personnel. It was decided to concentrate hospitals into groups. After taking numerous factors into consideration, such as French and English examples, the American lines of communication, French ports available for use by the American Army, and potentially available sites for hospitals, recommendations were approved by the commander in chief for the erection of "hospital centers."

Hospital centers were of two types:
1) those established in French buildings and
2) newly constructed barrack hospitals. When the armistice was signed, five centers were in operation in French buildings and fourteen in constructed barrack hospitals.

The design scheme called for these centers to have between two and twenty independent base hospitals and a convalescent camp operating under one administrative head. The larger centers were planned to accommodate between 30,000 and 36,000 patients. Each center included its own auxiliary activities such as Quartermaster and Medical Department depots, laundry, bakery, motor transport, electricity plant, military police, and headquarters detachments.

This system allowed for specialization among hospitals, including a center for tuberculosis and an orthopedic and psychopathic hospital, in addition to those used for general surgery and medicine. Highly skilled specialists were detailed as consultants on the staffs of the commanding officers to supervise the proper care of the sick and wounded. These specialists were reportedly "of the most skilled that America ha[d] produced, including many of the leading and most prominent surgeons, neurologists, orthopedists, internists, and bacteriologists, of our country." (*Surgeon General Report, 1919, pp. 1340–1341*)

(Opposite) *Sterilizing room at Base Hospital No. 23.*

"By 1917 the French and English had almost exhausted the supply of available buildings in France for hospitalization and the large influx of French and Belgian refugees from the devastated areas had made heavy demands upon any remaining reserve. The buildings which could be turned over to the Americans by the French at this time were not well suited to American hospital organization and methods. In many cases the offerings were inaccessible, in a condition of bad repair, without modern sanitary plumbing, and too small and scattered to be operated to advantage under the American system of hospitalization. School buildings, hotels, casernes, and French hospitals, while not well suited to hospital purposes, were operated as military hospitals with more or less success.

Hotels as hospitals had not only the objections of being hard to administer, extravagant in the requirement of personnel, but were otherwise not generally suited for hospital purposes because of the numerous halls, small rooms, and many stairs. Those available were very largely summer hotels without heating facilities, with insufficient water and very limited plumbing, were expensive to operate in that the rental was high, many alterations had to be made, damages were sustained to the furniture in being removed, and, when returned to the owners, complete restoration was required to be made under the French law.

Inasmuch as construction was unavoidably delayed, it was necessary to lease hotels in large numbers and operate them as hospitals in order that the sick and wounded of the fast arriving troops could be cared for, notwithstanding the many objections to their use." (*Surgeon General Report, 1919, p. 1338*)

❧❧

Base Hospitals 23, 36, 32, and 31 were assigned to the towns of Vittel and Contrexeville, and were originally equipped by the American Red Cross. These units arrived between November 1917 and January 1918, and formed the Vittel Hospital Center.

(Opposite) *Dressing room on the second floor at Base Hospital No. 23, Vittel, France.*

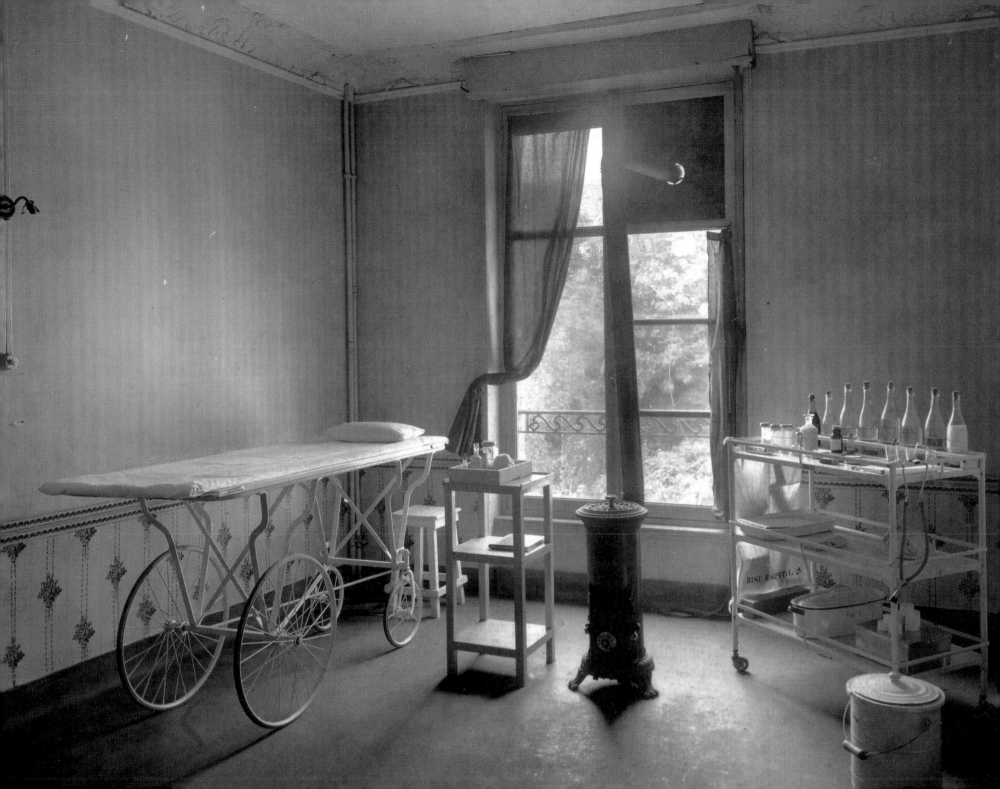

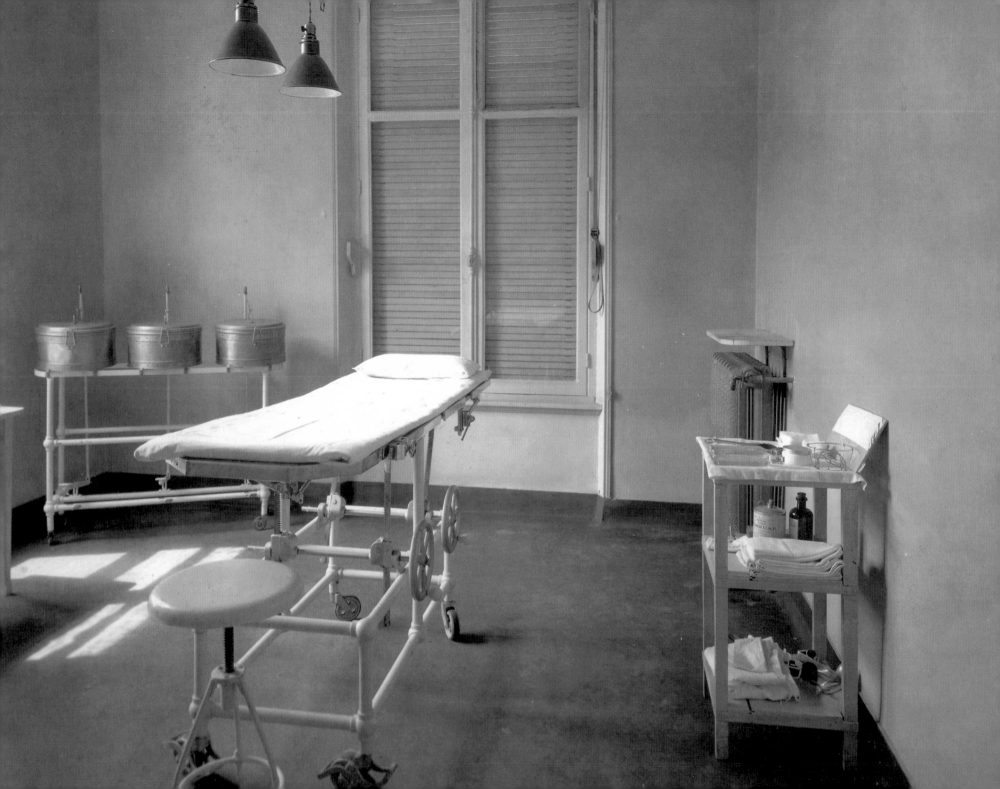

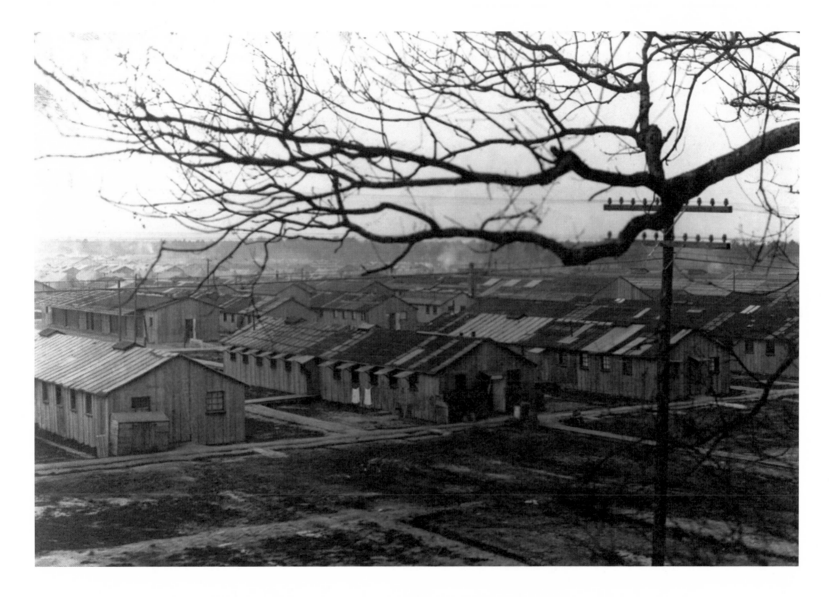

(Opposite) *Operating room No. 2 of Base Hospital No. 23, Hospital Center at Vittel. June 1918.*

(Above) *Aerial photograph of Evacuation Hospital No. 20, a component of the Beau Desert Hospital Center.*

"Beau Desert was selected as a hospital center for the AEF during the latter part of 1917 and work begun in December of that year. The site is a nearly level tract of land of approximately 550 acres and shaped something like a keystone." Beau Desert was formerly a hunting ground and had also been used for training horses and for races, and in some of the old buildings were found racing programs dating back many years. The area is nearly due west and approximately five miles from Bordeaux.

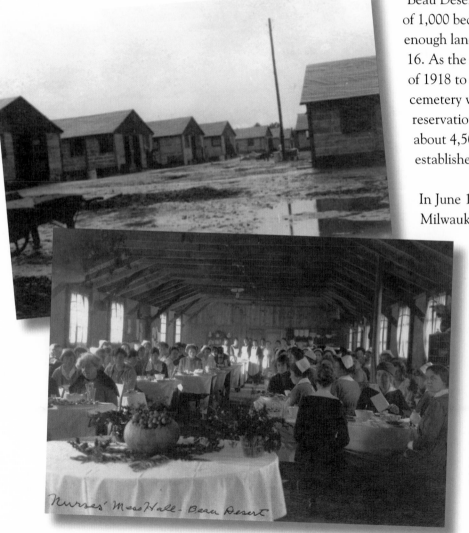

Nurses' Mess Hall - Beau Desert

"Beau Desert was originally selected as the site for 10 base hospitals of 1,000 beds each, with an emergency expansion to 1,500 each, but enough land was reserved to increase the number of hospitals to 16. As the war progressed, it became necessary during the summer of 1918 to complete an entire 17 units. As the center enlarged, a cemetery was added at the extreme southeastern portion of the reservation, and land was requisitioned for a convalescent camp of about 4,500 beds. In the fall of 1918, a farm and garden were also established." (*Surgeon General Report, 1919, p. 1855*)

In June 1918, Base Hospital No. 22, a Red Cross unit from Milwaukee, Wisconsin, and Base Hospital No. 114, organized at Allentown, Pennsylvania, arrived in France. On January 23, 1919, Base Hospital No. 22 ceased to function, and was ordered back to the United States to be mustered out of service. Evacuation Hospital No. 20, newly arrived from the Marne, where it had had only a few days' experience at the front, was ordered to take the place of No. 114. At the close of the war, the majority of the sick and wounded were evacuated through Beau Desert, thus changing the function of the hospital center to an evacuation center. Thereafter, Evacuation Hospital No. 20 was charged with the entire duty of evacuating patients and the hospital enlarged correspondingly to 2,500 beds. (*Surgeon General Report, 1919, p. 1858*)

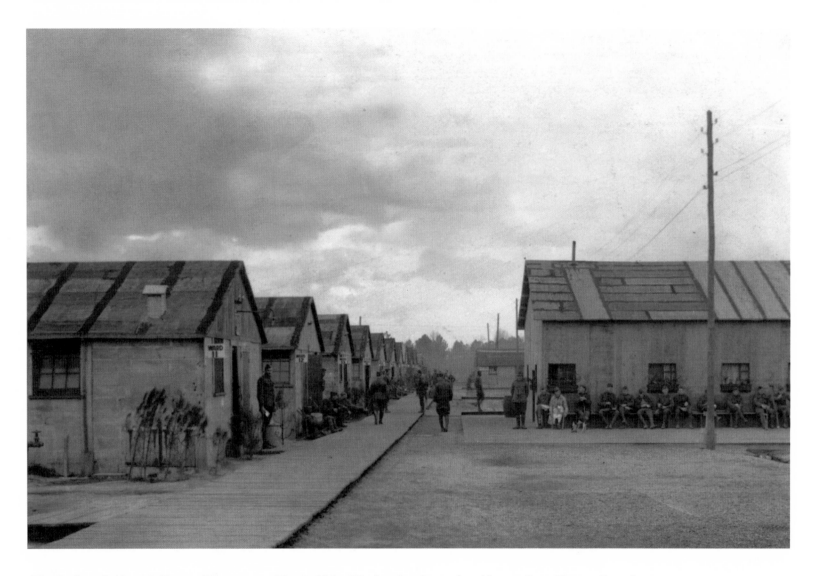

(Top Left and Above) *Views of Evacuation Hospital No. 20, showing the mud problem at Beau Desert. From here, all patients were evacuated from France to the United States.*

(Bottom Left) *Nurses' mess hall at Beau Desert Hospital Center, France.*

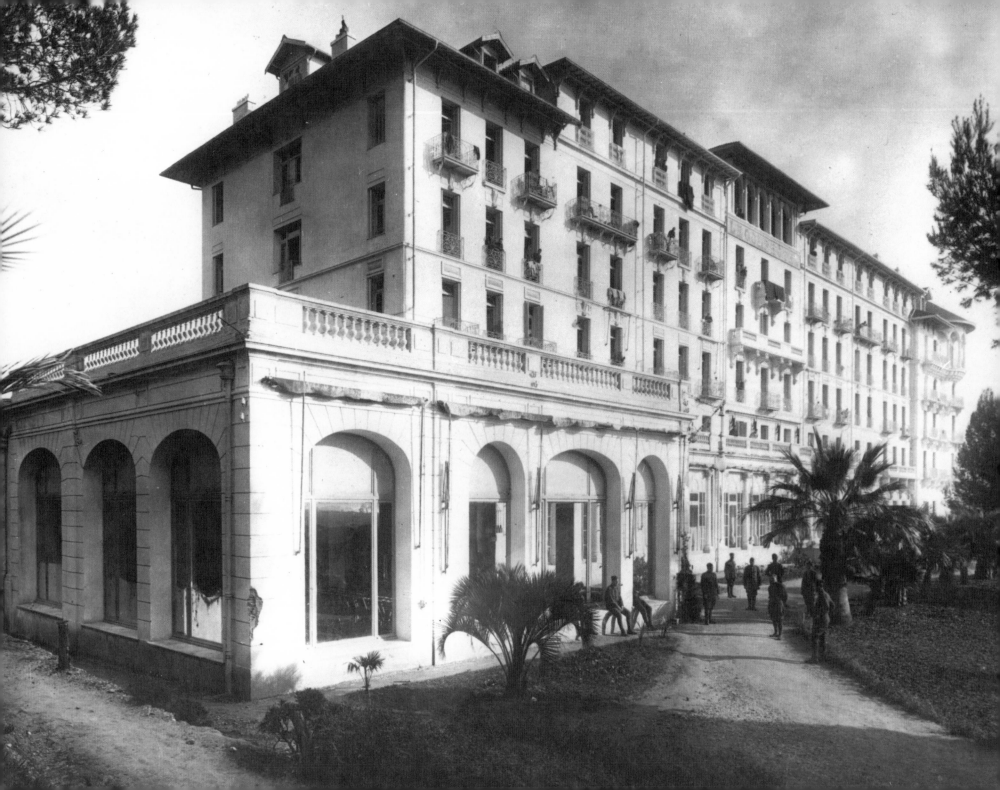

"The origin of the Riviera hospital center was an urgent need for a location for hospitals that would give the maximum hours of sunshine and clear skies, even temperature, and the most stimulating atmospheric conditions within practicable distance of the advanced areas. This was found in that strip of coast line extending from Marseille to Menton, called the Cote d'Azure, or Riviera." Here, facing the Mediterranean Sea and sheltered by the Maritime Alps, rainfall was limited and the climate mild rather than hot.

"It was too far from the scene of active operations to receive cases of recent injuries or acute illness, and therefore all cases received were patients who had so far recovered as to be able to stand a long journey. The center comprised all the hospitals along the north coast of the Mediterranean from Toulon to the Italian border, and functioned as a group of convalescent hospitals." *(Surgeon General Report, 1919, p. 1853)*

"Until shortly after the signing of the armistice there was no local member of the Nurse Corps who had supervisory control over all the nurses at one center. In order that the director of nursing service might keep more closely informed as to the nurses and their living and working conditions the plan was adopted of assigning center chief nurses to 11 of the large hospital centers. These center chief nurses were regarded as assistants to the director." Center chief nurse duties included assisting the commanding officer in matters involving the center's nurses "as he may see fit to assign to her" and "to act as hostess of the center." *(The Medical Dept in the World War, Vol. II, pp. 333–334)*

(Opposite) *Le Golf Hotel Hospital Center, Riviera. Group 1, Hyeres, consisted of nine hotels, with a total capacity of 3,600. This group was first designated Convalescent Hospital No. 1, but on arrival of Base Hospital No. 99, on November 26, 1918, its designation was changed to that of a base hospital.*

(Left) *Ward "O," the fracture ward in Base Hospital No. 115, Vichy Hospital Center.*

(Opposite) *In 1919, Vichy, France, was a growing popular summer resort known as "little Paris." Pictured here is the surgical ward in Base Hospital No. 1 (Bellevue Hospital Unit). The photograph shows the ward surgeon irrigating a wound of the right inguinal region accompanied by a nurse.*

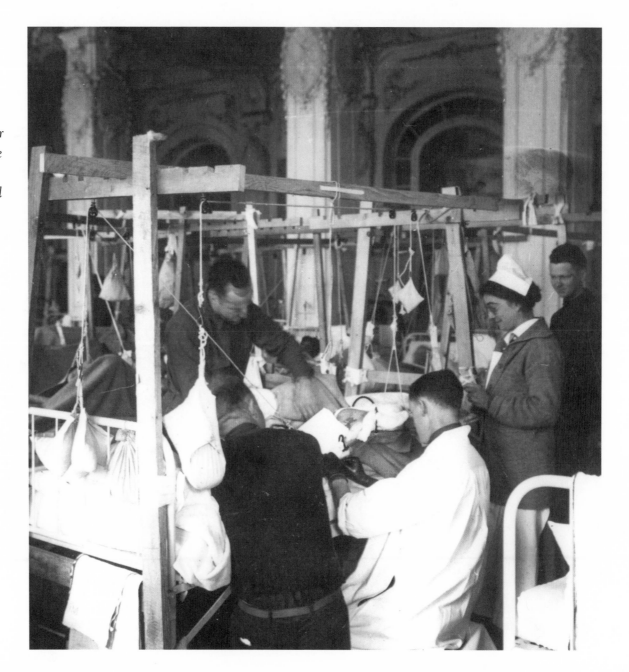

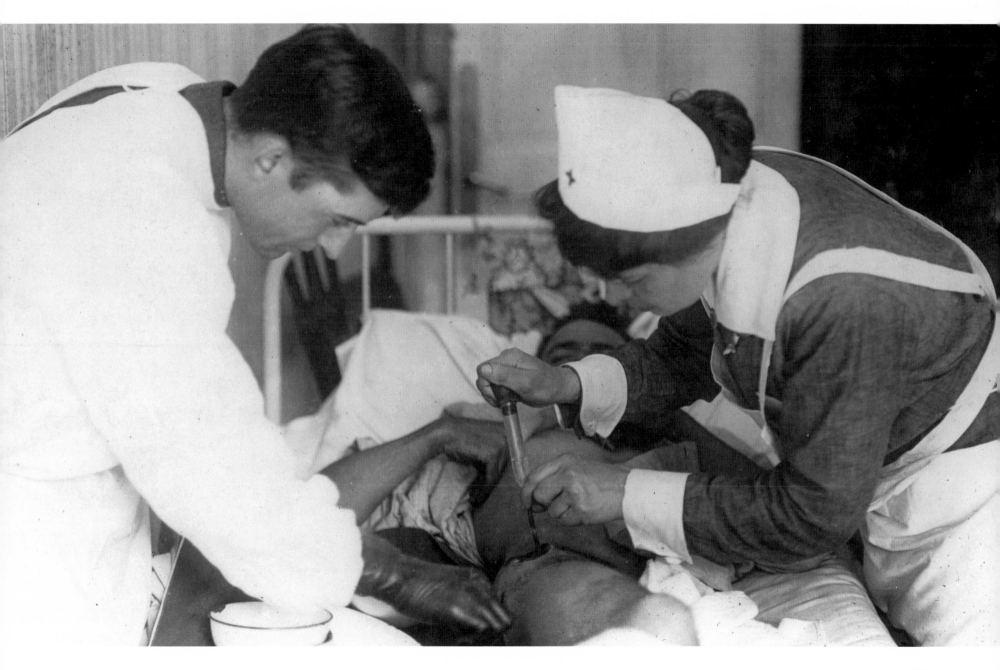

"The hospital center of Savenay was located in the city of that name, about 18 miles northeast of St. Nazaire. Its construction was authorized by the commander in chief in February, 1918. A convalescent camp was also authorized, with a capacity of 5,200 beds. The center was organized on August 5, 1918, when the commanding officer of Base Hospital No. 8 was also appointed commanding officer of the Savenay center. Several miles of standard-gauge track were constructed and spur tracks laid to connect the various units of the center and about a mile and a half of roads were built in the units. Each unit was connected by telephone with a central exchange, installed by the Signal Corps. Electric power was obtained from a French producer at St. Nazaire.

The location of Savenay, within one hour by rail of the port of St. Nazaire, and only seven hours from Brest, made it particularly important as an evacuation center. Prior to November 11, 1918, all AEF patients returned to the United States on surgeon's certificate of disability were evacuated through Savenay. Until that date efforts of the Medical Department were directed to sending men back to duty where possible, and large numbers of evacuations were made to the convalescent camp and from that camp back to duty." (*The Medical Dept in the World War, Vol. II, pp. 596–597*)

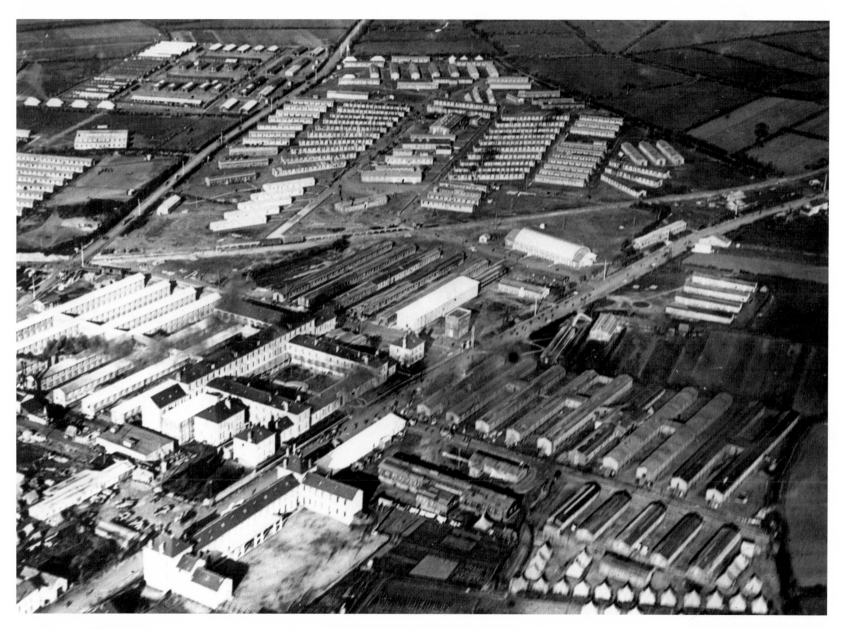

Aerial view of the Hospital Center at Savenay, France. Undated.

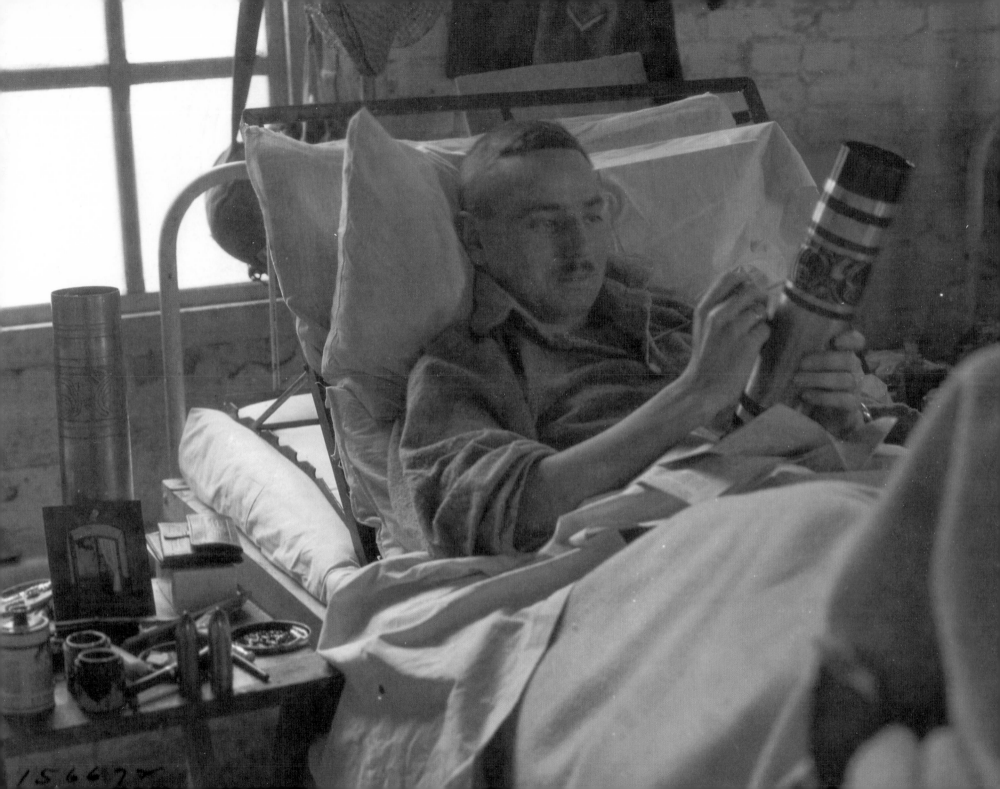

15-667

Convalescence

On August 21, 1918, orders were received from the chief surgeon's office to establish a convalescent camp as a unit separate from the hospital at Savenay. In compliance, a site was selected where the parade ground measured approximately 1,800 by 600 feet. Fifty pyramidal tents were put up and 300 French beds placed in the tents for use by the patients. This change from hospital to convalescent camp was made in one day, and the patients were transferred from hospital to camp. *(The Medical Dept in the World War, Vol. II, pp. 596–600)*

"It is not generally realized what an important function a convalescent camp may play with regard to the return of the soldiers from the hospitals to duty. And the function is not only that of returning men to duty, but primarily is concerned with the revitalizing of troops. Consequently, the more completely that soldiers are allowed to rest their minds from the worries incident to battle, the keener the spirit they will manifest upon being thrown into battle the second time. This mental rest is best accomplished by light duties, entertainment, and interesting occupations." *(Surgeon General Report, 1919, p. 2149)*

(Opposite) *Sergeant William Waterman, Co. A, 348th Machine Gun Battalion, 91st Division, wounded in the right hip on September 27, 1918, in the Argonne. Waterman is decorating shells during his convalescence at Base Hospital No. 69, Savenay.*

(Right) *Nurse P.E. Walters cheers patients Private Tuties and Sergeant Howard, during their convalescence at a base hospital in France. Location unknown.*

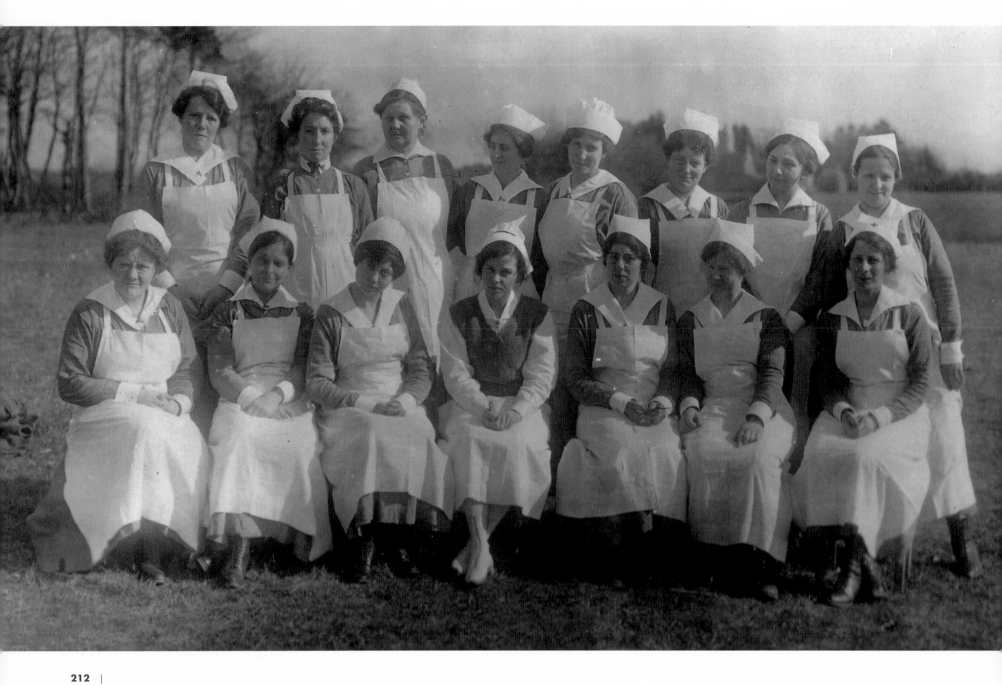

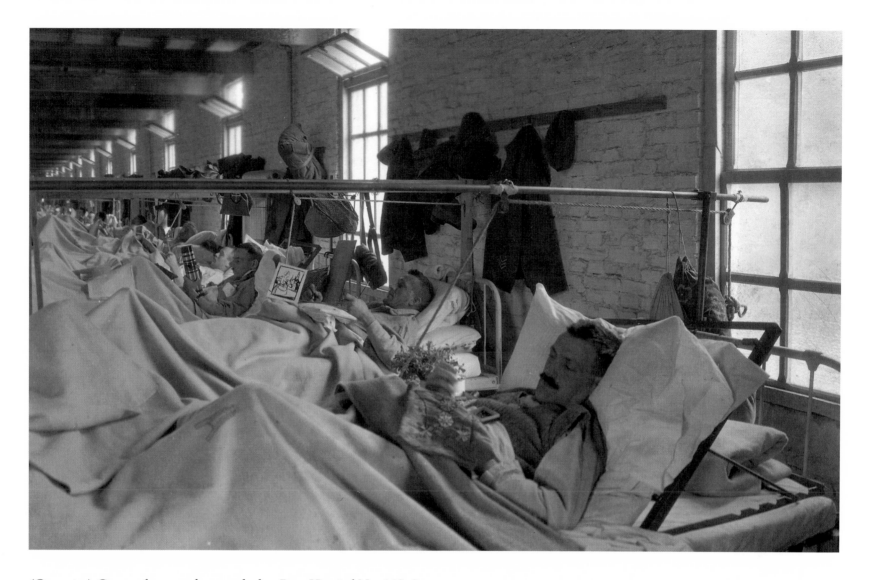

(Opposite) *Group of nurses photographed at Base Hospital No. 118, Savenay.*

(Above) *Patients primarily from the 91st and 1st Divisions are shown confined to bed but engaged in what were considered "useful" activities, such as decorating shells and bead work.*

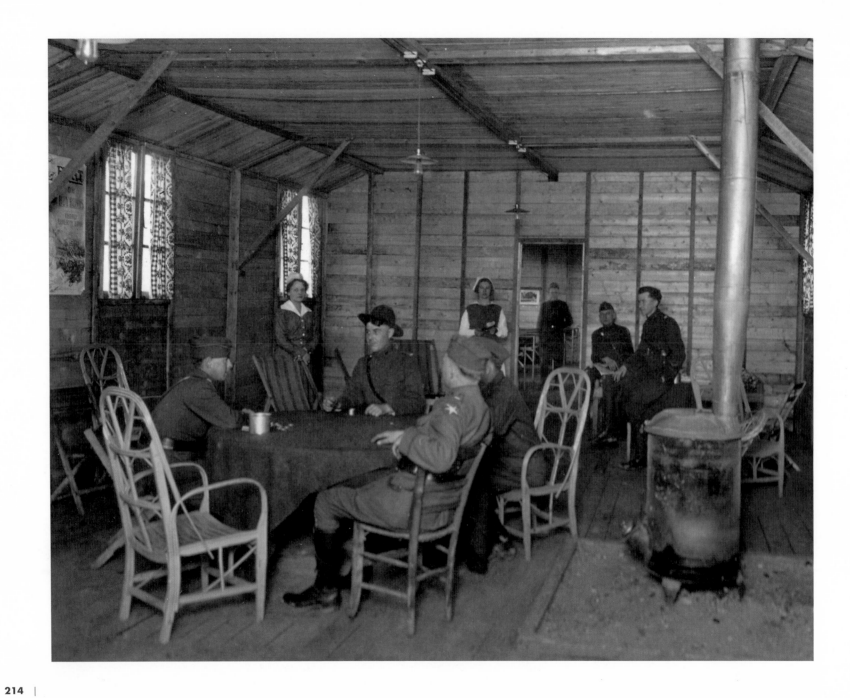

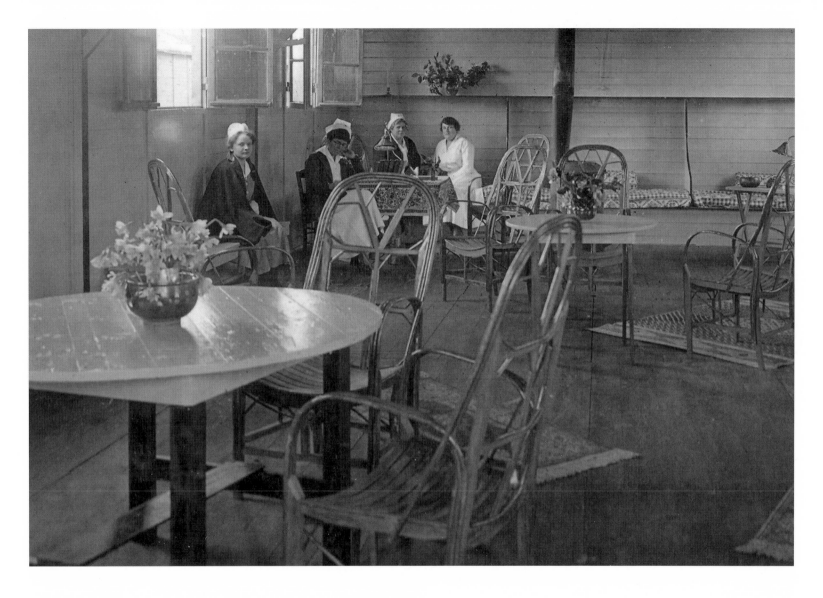

(Opposite) *Officers' recreation hut, Base Hospital No. 214 at Savenay.*

(Above) *Nurses' recreation hut, Base Hospital No. 214 at Savenay.*

Victory!

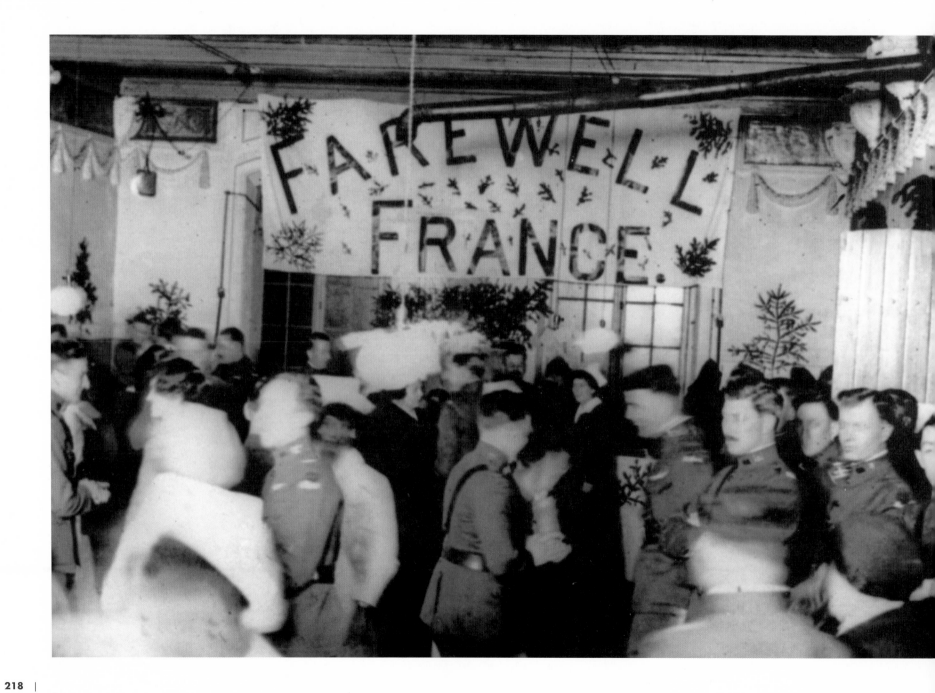

Farewell to France

"NOVEMBER 11, 1918: MONDAY—The Armistice has been signed, for sure this time. The beginning of the end of this awful war. Everyone was officially requested to remain sane, no demonstration as of last Friday, no drinking!

When the news became official at 11 AM the Mayor, through the town Crier, declared a Holiday, flags were immediately displayed and there was much rejoicing and many tears were shed. [Some of] the local people were sick at heart to realize their sons would never return. Our firing squad fired the twenty-one volleys as an Honorary Salute. The Mayor kissed Col. Clark on both cheeks, and their was much hand shaking, no shouting, no band and very little drinking, many of the local homes, lawns doorways and roofs are decorated with colored lights and the whole town was lighted for the first time since our arrival. Everything looks festive, I was on duty, all day but made some divinity [fudge] in evening to celebrate." *(Maude Frances Essig)*

❧❦

"During the first portion of the war, nurses were not allowed to socialize with enlisted men. In the spring of 1919, the policy inexplicably changed. Stimson reported that 'the result was well-nigh disastrous.' At one embarkation center . . . at Vannes, the nurses were so overwhelmed with enlisted men's attentions that they requested an immediate reinstatement of the ban forbidding fraternization between enlisted men and nurses. In May 1919, it was reinstated and 'no further trouble was experienced.'" *(Sarnecky, p. 117)*

(Opposite) *Farewell party at Base Hospital No. 45.*

La Baule and St. Nazaire

"To facilitate the return of nurses to the United States, beginning in January, 1919, Camp Hospital No. 91, La Baule, functioned as a centralization point for the Army Nurse Corps under orders to return to the United States. The location was chosen because La Baule is a seaside resort not far from the Savenay Hospital Center and the port of St. Nazaire, and but a short distance by train from Brest. The nurses who were sent to La Baule to prepare for return to the United States were housed in four large hotels, built of brick or stone, of excellent construction, but without arrangements for central heating.

The average length of stay for the units at La Baule was from 10 to 15 days, as it required much time to complete the records and make arrangements for the journey to the United States. Frequently, the four hotels were taxed by the many units reporting there simultaneously. Entertainment was provided by the American Red Cross and also by the administrative staff of the hospital in the form of bus rides to St. Nazaire, auto trips, dances twice a week, and moving-picture shows." *(The Medical Dept in the World War, Vol. XIII, p. 347)*

(Opposite) *Nurses' dining room at the Hotel Royal, La Baule, Loire Inferieure, France.*

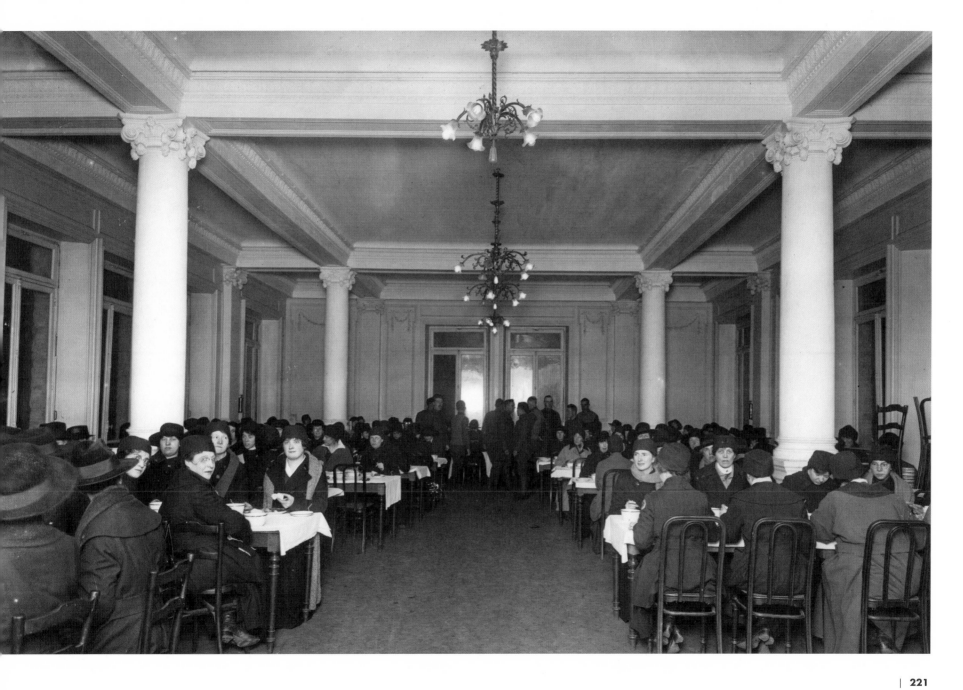

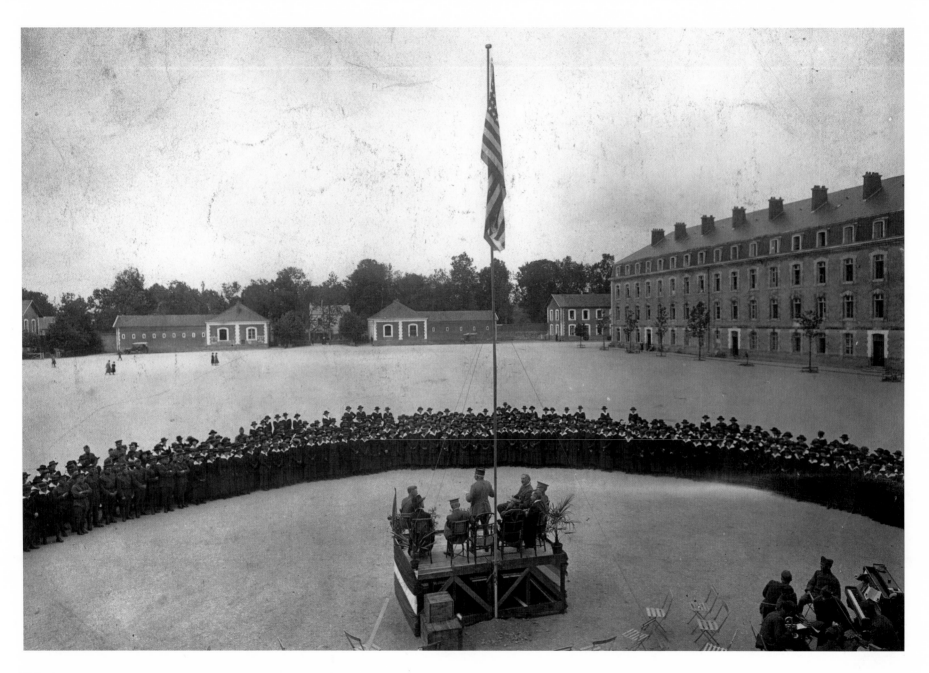

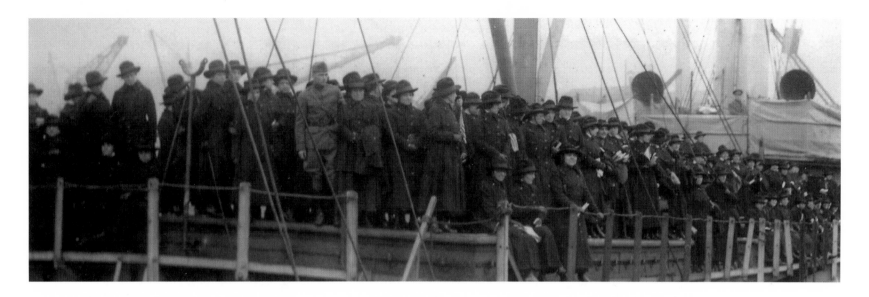

"Another important concentration camp for nurses was at the Vannes Hospital Center. At Vannes the one hospital, Base Hospital No. 136, was in old French buildings which formed three sides of a quadrangle and which previously had been French barracks. The buildings were very dirty and required an unusual amount of work to convert them into a decently liveable place. There were no proper toilet arrangements, no electricity, and gas in but a few of the buildings. The only advantages of the place were an abundance of room, plenty of potable water, and freedom from mud. This hospital was the nucleus of the center. On May 30, 1919, there were 1,157 nurses at Vannes awaiting orders to return to the United States." *(The Medical Dept in the World War, p. 348)*

(Opposite) *General Foch and other dignitaries speaking before a large group of nurses preparing for departure to the United States during Memorial Day services at Vannes, France, 1919.*

(Above) *The Signal Corps photograph caption states: "Nurses of 30th Hospital Unit on board transport at Brest, France. May 5, 1918." [probably Base Hospital 30]*

Awards and Citations

In the summer of 1918 the War Department gave ANC members the authority to wear wound and service chevrons under the same conditions as officers, field clerks, and enlisted men. Nurses who served honorably in the Army Nurse Corps for a minimum of 15 days during a period of the war were entitled to the Victory "Button," issued for wear in the lapel of civilian clothes.

"For their exceptional service during the period of the war, three Army nurses received the Distinguished Service Cross. The Army recognized the contributions of twenty-five other Army nurses with the Distinguished Service Medal. France bestowed the *Croix de Guerre* on twenty-eight members of the Army Nurse Corps and Great Britain acknowledged sixty-nine American Army nurses with the British Royal Red Cross and gave two the British Military Medal." *(Sarnecky, p. 131)*

❧❧

"We have been officially notified to provide ourselves with service strips (2) for our one year of foreign service; 'V' gold to be worn on our left sleeve just above the cuff." *(January 19, 1919, Maude Frances Essig)*

(Opposite) *Nurses of Base Hospital No. 41 wearing new service stripes on their sleeves, on board USS Cartago, St. Nazaire. March 18, 1919.*

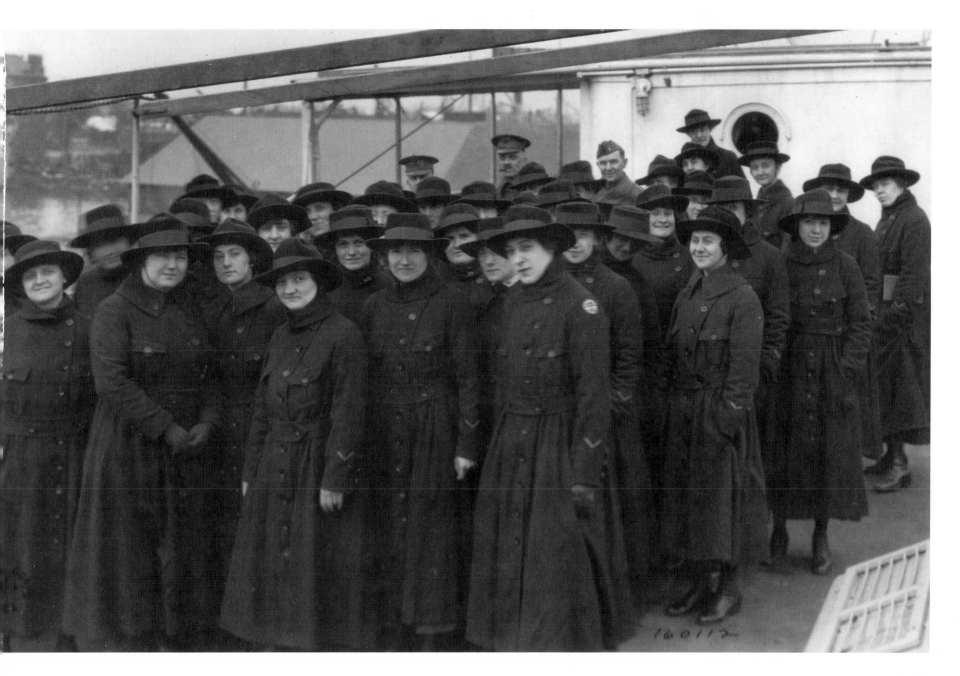

The War of 1914–1918.

American Nursing Corps.

Nurse Miss H. G. McClelland. Philadelphia Unit.

was mentioned in a Despatch from

Field Marshal Sir Douglas Haig. K.T. G.C.B. G.C.V.O. K.C.I.E.

dated 7th November 1917

for gallant and distinguished services in the Field.

I have it in command from the King to record His Majesty's

high appreciation of the services rendered.

Winston S. Churchill

War Office
Whitehall. S.W.
1st March 1919.

Secretary of State for War.

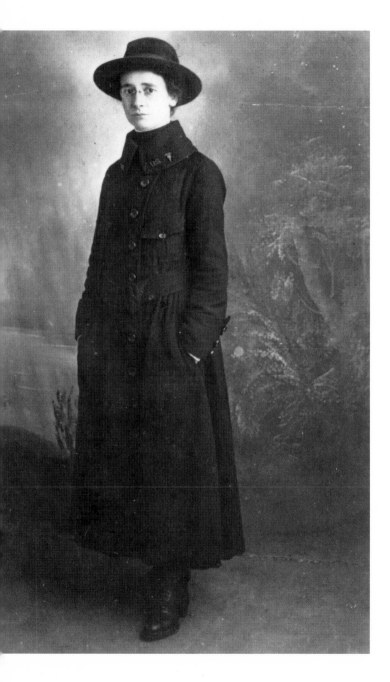

Distinguished Service Cross

Possibly the most decorated woman in military service to date, Helen Grace McClelland of Fredericktown, Ohio, was a graduate of the Pennsylvania Hospital School of Nursing. McClelland served as a reserve nurse with the Army Nurse Corps in France and Belgium for Base Hospital No. 10, where her distinguished service on the front lines earned her a citation from General Sir Douglas Haig, the Royal Red Cross First Class from Britain, and the Distinguished Service Medal and Distinguished Service Cross from the United States.

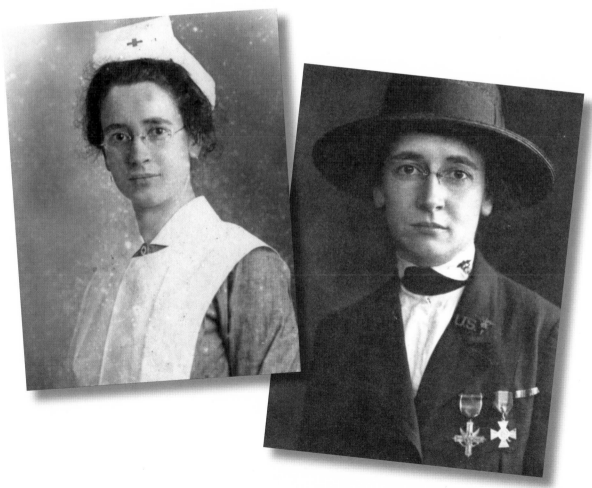

The Distinguished Service Cross is the nation's second highest military decoration. The first army nurse to be awarded the Distinguished Service Cross was Beatrice MacDonald.

In July 1917, MacDonald left the comfort and safety of her unit, Evacuation Hospital No. 2, to move forward on the battlefield as a member of a small surgical team to augment the British No. 61 Casualty Clearing Station, operating in the British area at the time. On the night of August 17, MacDonald was awakened by bombs. While reaching for her tin hat, she was struck by shrapnel in the right eye and cheek. Her tent mate, Helen McClelland, immediately began to care for her. MacDonald was placed on a stretcher, taken to the operating tent, and later transferred to the ophthalmic center in Boulogne. (During World War I, before high-speed evacuation and treatment were available, convalescence from devastating injuries was conducted in theater.) After her recovery, MacDonald, now sightless in her right eye, returned to duty. She remained in Boulogne and assumed chief nurse duties at Evacuation Hospital No. 2 for nine months, until January 1919.

Upon returning from the war, MacDonald was called to Congress, and received the Distinguished Service Cross on February 27, 1919. (Helen McClelland also received the Distinguished Service Cross for her actions that day.)

(Opposite) *Beatrice MacDonald, post-injury, in France.*

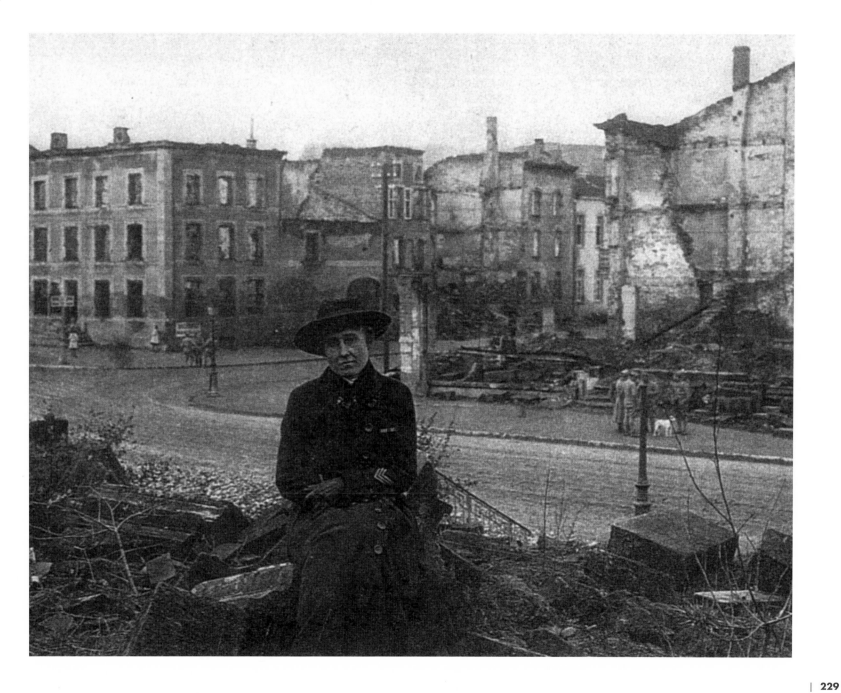

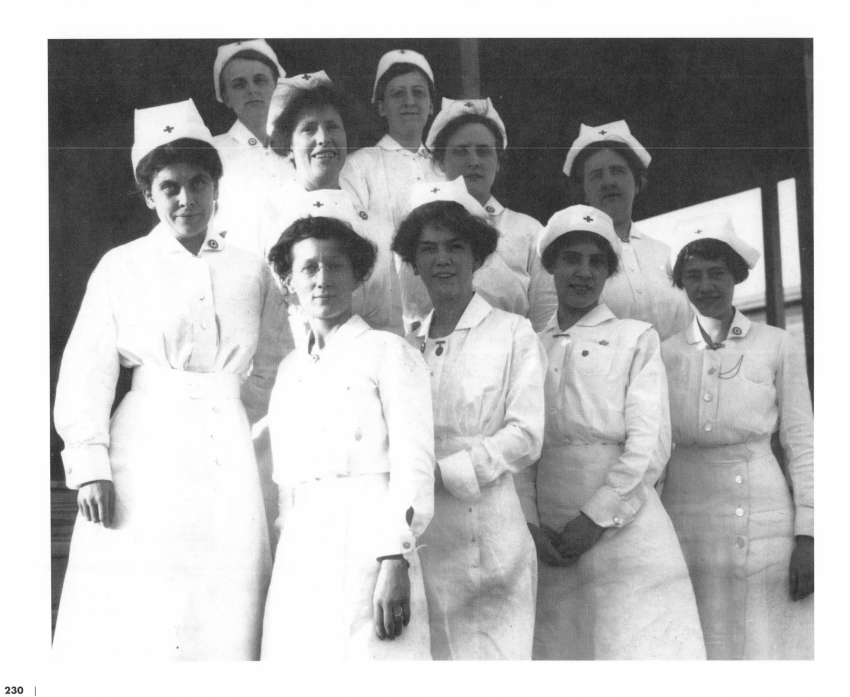

"Isabel Stambaugh, Reserve Nurse, Army Nurse Corps, Base Hospital No. 10 (Philadelphia) while with a surgical team at a British Casualty Clearing Station during the German drive of March 21, 1918, in front of Amiens, France, was seriously wounded by shell fire from German aeroplanes." *(Distinguished Service Cross General Order no. 70)*

Stambaugh was a graduate of the Presbyterian Hospital, Philadelphia, Pennsylvania, and later served for two years as head operating nurse at the same hospital.

Stambaugh served with one of the six U.S. hospitals lent to the British army. She saw most of her service in the evacuation hospital (known as a clearing station to the British army) at Le Treport, behind the Somme sector in France. On March 21, 1918, a shell dropped in the operating room where Stambaugh, a surgeon, and an anaesthetist were working. She was cited by Field Marshal Haig for bravery under fire and was later awarded the Distinguished Service Cross.

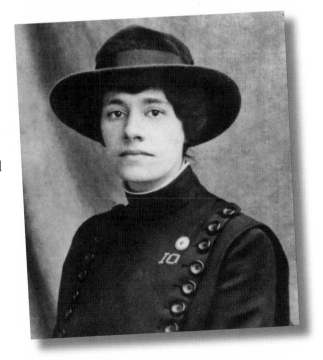

Silver Star Medal (formerly Citation Star)

During the latter months of World War I, the Citation Star was authorized by Congress to be conferred for gallantry under enemy fire. It consisted of a small (3/16-in. in diameter) silver star device worn on the World War I Victory Medal. In 1932, the Citation Star became the Silver Star Medal. Three World War I Army Nurses were the first known women to receive the Citation Star.

(Opposite) *Isabel Stambaugh [pictured on the far left] with other Red Cross Nurses, date and place unknown.*

(Right) *Isabel Stambaugh in uniform.*

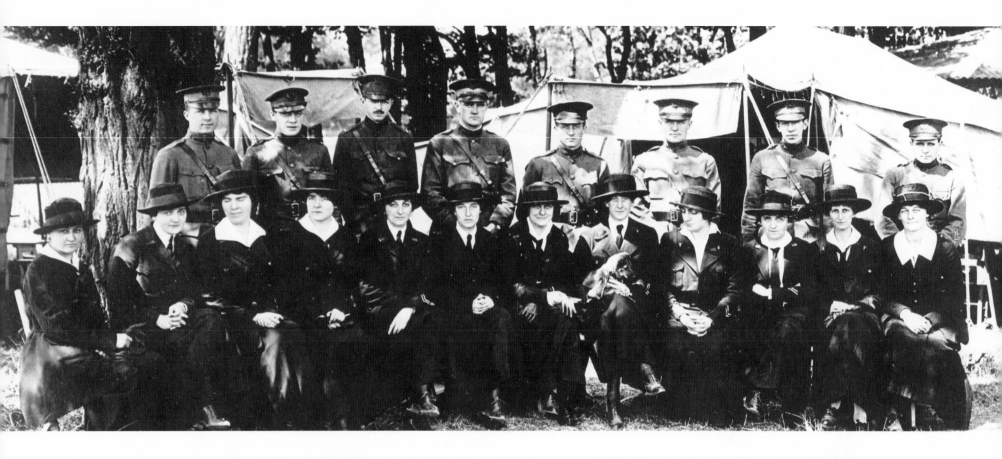

Jane I. Rignel, the chief nurse of Mobile Hospital No 2, was awarded the Citation Star for gallantry in "giving aid to the wounded soldiers under heavy enemy fire" on July 15, 1918, in Bussey-le-Chateau, France. Despite heavy artillery fire that destroyed parts of the hospital, Rignel and other staff continued providing patient care at the front.

(Above) *Jane I. Rignel (holding dog), chief nurse of Mobile Hospital No. 2, was awarded the Citation Star for gallantry in July 1918.*

(Opposite) *The certificate awarding the Citation Star to Linnie Leckrone, Army Nurse Corps, for gallantry in battle, signed by AEF Commander-in-Chief General John Pershing. Female pronouns were used so infrequently in this document that the clerk simply lined through the male ones.* (Photograph courtesy of Mary Jane Bolles-Reed)

The two other recipients, Linnie E. Leckrone and Irene Robar, both of the Army Nurse Corps, were attached to Field Hospital No. 127. They were awarded the Citation Star for gallantry while "attending to the wounded during [an] artillery bombardment" on July 29, 1918, in Chateau-Thierry France. Leckrone and Robar were volunteer members of a six-person shock team that provided resuscitative care to trauma patients by augmenting a forwardly deployed hospital.

The three women likely never knew the significance of their awards, for the Citation Star was usually posted in orders over a year after the event and never formerly presented to the recipients. In 1932 all three women were authorized to exchange their Citation Stars for the Silver Star Medal in a paperwork process that was considered a formality. In July 2007, the acting Surgeon General of the U.S. Army presented the Silver Star Medal to the daughter of Linnie Leckrone, Mary Jane Bolles-Reed.

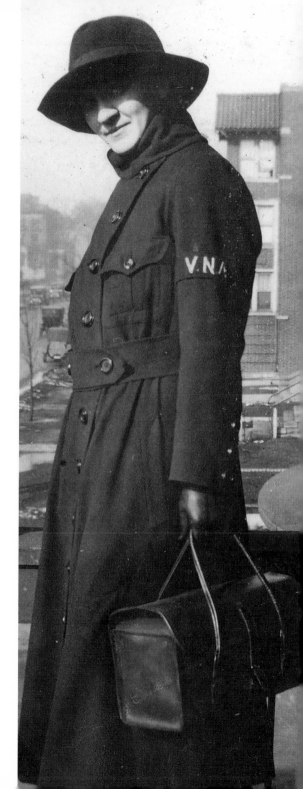

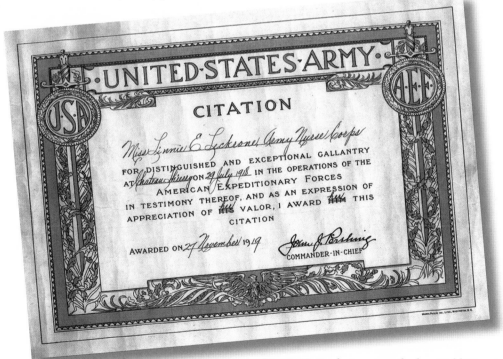

Linnie E. Leckrone, attached to Field Hospital No. 127, who was awarded the Citation Star for gallantry in July 1918.

Irene Robar, Army Nurse Corps, attached to Field Hospital No. 127, was awarded the Citation Star for gallantry while tending to the wounded during an artillery bombardment on July 29, 1918.

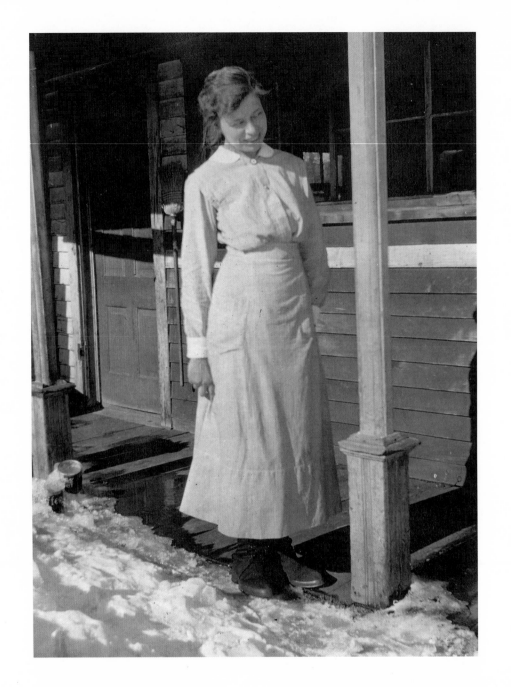

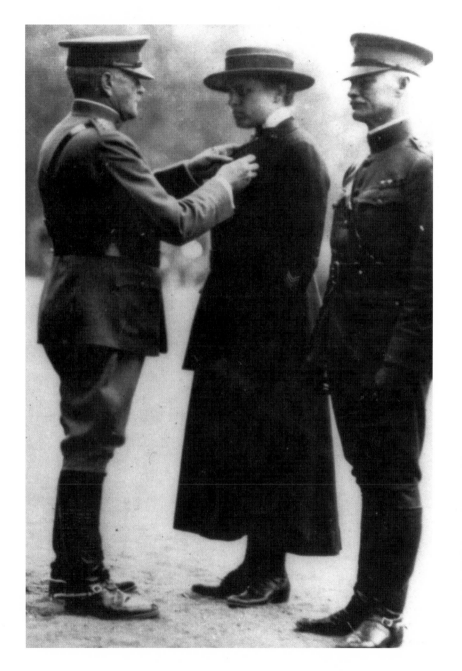

Distinguished Service Medal

"Stimson was recognized by the United States, Great Britain, and France for her tireless efforts during the war, which contributed to reduced mortality rates in military hospitals. She was awarded the American Distinguished Service Medal; the British Royal Red Cross, 1st Class; the French *Médaille de la Reconnaissance Française*; the *Médaille d'Hygiéne Publique*; and the International Red Cross Florence Nightingale Medal for her services during the war and recovery period." *(Pocklington, p. 32)*

(Left and Below) Julia C. Stimson, Chief of Army Nurse Corps, *being decorated with the Distinguished Service Medal by General John J. Pershing, Tours, France. June 5, 1919.*

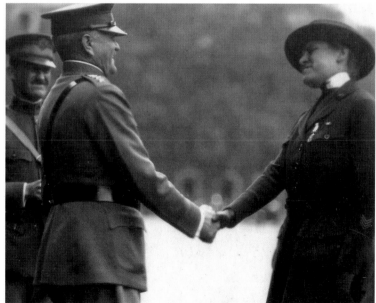

Summary

ON THE DAY THE ARMISTICE WAS SIGNED, November 11, 1918, there were in the service, or under orders to proceed to their first station, 3,524 regular nurses and 17,956 reserve nurses, making a total of 21,480. All were experienced professional women who volunteered to serve a draftee army.

Army nurses came from all over the United States to take care of their brothers and neighbors. Twenty years earlier, during the Spanish-American War, nurses were kept safe in camps far from the lines, but by 1918 nurses sought out service on the front lines. With little idea of the conditions they would face, these brave and dedicated nurses proved themselves capable of acting heroically under fire, as well as serving essential roles as members of healthcare teams whose dedication and skills significantly reduced the morbidity and mortality rates of the soldiers in their care. Although remaining largely unrewarded for their service, the accomplishments of World War I nurses would forever change the Army Nurse Corps.

When the influenza pandemic peaked in 1918, nurses were asked yet again to serve in hospitals across the nation, providing care for those stricken and training the next generation of nurses. By the war's end in 1918, the total capacity of the 153 base hospitals, 66 camp hospitals, and 12 convalescent camps operating was 192,844 normal and 276,347 emergency beds, of which 184,421 were occupied.

The 1920s brought Army nurses a rudimentary rank system endorsed by the Army leadership, the soldiers they cared for, the Army Medical Department, and the civilian nursing community. From 1918 on, military nurses were an essential element in the provision of medical care at the front.

Acknowledgements

THIS PHOTOGRAPHIC COLLECTION WOULD NOT HAVE BEEN POSSIBLE without the assistance of a supportive, cheerful, and knowledgeable team of collaborators. Within the Office of Medical History a special word of thanks goes to Lt. Col. Richard Prior for his patient technical advice and skill, an in-depth awareness of Army Nurse Corps history during the World War I period, and a "can do" attitude that made working with him a true pleasure. Thanks also go to my colleagues Dr. John Greenwood and Dr. Sanders Marble, for lending a hand with their historical wisdom and proofreading.

Outside our offices, Emily A. Court, MLS, of the Armed Forces Medical Library, managed to secure a wealth of hard-to-find publications and research information for us. We thank her for contributing such time and effort on our behalf.

Lastly, we extend our appreciation to the following: The Army Heritage Center Foundation at Carlisle, Pennsylvania, for the loan of material on Elizabeth Lewis; Nelle Fairchild Hefty Rote for her archival donations and permission to quote from her book *Nurse Helen Fairchild*; Quannah Santiago for donating the Grand Hotel Beau-Site brochure from Aix-les-Bains; Myrna Babineau for the photograph of Beatrice MacDonald, and the Navy Bureau of Medicine and Surgery Archives for the photograph of Esther V. Hasson.

Bibliography

ESSIG, MAUDE FRANCES. *My Trip Abroad With Uncle Sam— 1917-1919. American Expeditionary Forces in France, Reserve Army Nurse Corps, American Red Cross Nurse #4411 ("How We Won World War I")*. Undated. Photocopied collection in Army Nurse Corps Archives, Office of Medical History, The Office of the Surgeon General, Falls Church, VA.

GAVIN, LETTIE. *American Women in World War I; They Also Served.* (University Press of Colorado: Boulder, CO, 1997).

IRELAND, MAJOR GENERAL M.W. *The Medical Department of the United States Army in the World War.* (U.S. Government Printing Office: Washington, D.C., 1927).

LUCIANO, LORRAINE AND CASANDRA JEWELL. *Army Nurses of World War One, Service Beyond Expectations.* (Army Heritage Center Foundation: Carlisle, PA, 2006).

MACPHERSON, MAJOR-GENERAL SIR W.G. *History of the Great War: Medical Services General History, Vol. II.* (London: His Majesty's Stationery Office, 1923).

Pennsylvania Hospital Unit in the Great War. (Paul B. Hoebert: New York, NY, 1921)

POCKLINGTON, DOROTHY B. *Heritage of Leadership, Army Nurse Corps Biographies.* (Aldot Publishing House: Ellicott City, MD, 2004).

Report of the Surgeon General U.S. Army to the Secretary of War, 1919, Vol. II. (Government Printing Office: Washington, D.C., 1919).

RIECKE, JOCOBINA R. *Diary of Miss Jocobina R. Riecke During World War I.* Undated. Photocopied collection in Army Nurse Corps Archives, Office of Medical History, The Office of the Surgeon General, Falls Church, VA.

ROTE, NELLE FAIRCHILD *Nurse Helen Fairchild WW1, 1917-1918.* (Fisher Fairchild Publishing Co.: Lewisburg, PA, 2004).

SARNECKY, MARY T. *A History of the U.S. Army Nurse Corps.* (University of Pennsylvania Press: Philadelphia, PA, 1999).

STIMSON, JULIA C. *Finding Themselves.* (The Macmillan Company: NY, 1918).

WIGLE, SHARI LYNN. *Pride of America, The Letters of Grace Anderson U.S. Army Nurse Corps, World War I.* (Seaboard Press: Rockville, MD, 2007).